Traditional Native Leadership
~ The 10 Scrolls ~

Also by Don L. Coyhis

Alcohol Problems in Native America:
The Untold Story of Resistance and Recovery–
"The Truth About the Lie"

Don L. Coyhis & William L. White,
2006

Meditations with Native American Elders:
The Four Seasons

Don L. Coyhis
2007

Understanding the Purpose of Life:
12 Teachings for Native Youth

Don L. Coyhis
2008

Understanding Native American Culture:
Insights for Recovery Professionals
and Other Wellness Practitioners

Don L. Coyhis
Edited by Richard Simonelli
2009

The Wellbriety Movement Comes of Age:
The Fulfillment of Prophecy

Don L. Coyhis
Edited by Richard Simonelli
2011

Traditional Native Leadership

The Ten Scrolls

Don L. Coyhis

Coyhis Publishing & Consulting, Inc.
Colorado Springs, Colorado

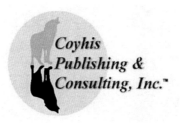

ISBN   978-1-5323-0348-7

Book design and layout by Richard Simonelli

1. Native American leadership and governance; 2. Native American health and healing; 3. Native American wisdom; 4. Native studies; 5. American studies.

To order books:

Coyhis Publishing Inc.
4775 Ford Drive
Colorado Springs, CO 80908

Toll-free 1-866-518-5275
303-363-9090
Fax: 303-856-7711
www.coyhispublishing.com
info@coyhispublishing.com

Dedication

This Native leadership book is dedicated to one of our council of Elders, Dr. Henrietta Mann, a beautiful and powerful Cheyenne Woman. She has spent her life dedicated to the betterment of Native people, Native sobriety, healthy Native women, men and families, and education. Some of the most visible people are the ones who try to help others in secret. The more they "hide," the more visible they are. Our Elder has been guiding and helping the Wellbriety Movement for many years. I cannot recall a time that she ever told us, *no, I have other plans.* We have been guided over the years and are grateful that the Creator has spoken to us through this wonderful, spiritual, traditional Native woman.

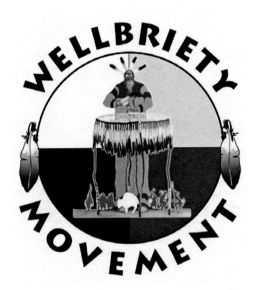

Foreword

All human beings, like all snowflakes, are unique. Yet once in a while in life you come across one who is unique in a way that it is clear the Creator had something special in mind. Don Coyhis is one of these.

I met Don in the mid 1970's and at that time we shared a common passion....drinking! Little did I know that our shared drinking misadventures would lead to both of us getting sober in 1978. As time went by we shared a commitment to serving others, a close and enduring friendship of nearly 40 years, and my being witness to how the Creator selected and used one individual to channel love and healing to Indigenous people and to alcoholics.

It seems to me that Don was being progressively reawakened to his Native American spiritual heritage and given access to an ever increasing amount of ancient wisdom–but on the understanding that he had to share it with everyone who could benefit from it. The story of how this resulted in the founding of the nonprofit *White Bison Inc.* and creation of *The Wellbriety Movement* has already been told in a previous book, "The Wellbriety Movement Comes of Age." I feel incredibly privileged to have been present to witness the birth and ongoing expansion of this Movement and know that it is still, after 25+ years, in an early stage of its ongoing healing work.

This brings me to one of the many reasons I find my old friend Don Coyhis to be an unusually unique human being. I personally don't know anyone else who has started and sustained a Movement that has so positively impacted the lives of thousands of people like the Wellbriety Movement has. I also know that he has always seen himself as a servant to this Movement rather than the director of it. This is a perfect example of *servant leadership* in action.

Now I am extremely excited to see this new book on leadership, which Don has been working on for some time, published and available to anyone who has an interest in the topic. Like some of his previous books this one is packed with a mixture of ancient wisdom and practical techniques for today's leaders in all cultures and walks of life. You will find many valuable tools and lessons presented in this story of Native American Leadership rediscovered. I hope you'll find the nuggets of leadership wisdom the Creator has channeled through author Don Coyhis, specifically for you.

Happy reading!

Wayne Records
White Bison, Inc. co-founder,
Former Board of Directors Chairman

Contents

Introduction

In the old days, the Ancient Ones had spiritual powers. Today, we would consider those powers to be special or exceptional.

In those days, they were normal. People were closely connected to nature and to the Creator. It was common for them to "see" into the future. It was common for the people to communicate with the animals and the other relatives of nature. This ability to see, and then pass this knowledge on to later generations is what we call prophecy. This gift to "see" and tell these stories from generation to generation gives our current generation hope and the knowledge to make decisions so we can lead our people. This process is called prophecy. The Elders spoke about what they knew to be true.

The Prophecy

The people will spend a long time in a cold winter. During this time, they will suffer. It will be a difficult time, a time of suffering, difficulty and confusion.

When the sun is blocked in the seventh moon, that wintertime will be over. The people will enter a new springtime, a time of brotherhood, a time of coming together.

When the springtime of healing begins, Mother Earth will distribute the powers and secrets of healing to the Native Women.

A sign will appear in the north. A white buffalo calf will be born as a sign to all people on the earth that we must now come together. We must change ourselves and accept all Earth people as our brothers and sisters. We are all related.

A white buffalo calf will be born in the north. It will turn four colors — red, yellow, black, and white. After the first calf is born, there will be three more, one for each of the four directions.

The young people will have old spirits.

A spider will build a web around Mother Earth. This web will carry our voice around the world to all nations.

When the healing time comes, an Eagle will land on the moon and return to Earth.

The White Buffalo Calf

In 1994 a white buffalo calf was born near Janesville, Wisconsin. This birth had an instant effect on the whole world. Native people from all over North America gathered to get a glimpse of the white buffalo calf. Many ceremonies were done and many of the Native Elders came forward with information about the meaning of the calf.

The white buffalo calf is the sign mentioned in the prophecy. This is the time of change in Indian communities. At this time we are to prepare ourselves to take our place as the teachers of the Earth. This is the time for the women to come forward. This is the time for Indian youth to become agents of change in our communities. This is the time for our Indian leaders to heal themselves. This is the beginning of the healing time foretold in our prophecies. It is a time of great urgency. The Hopi prophecies talk about three great shakings, warnings to human beings to align their thinking with the universal principles, laws, and values. We humans are to work together for unity and harmony. If we don't, the Creator is going to give us three warnings. The first Great Shaking was World War I, the second great shaking was World War II. In the third Great Shaking, it is said that Mother Earth will flip on her axis. This will happen if we humans don't start honoring the Creator's ways.

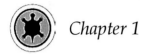 *Chapter 1*

The Wisdomkeepers

A long time ago, before the White Man came to Turtle Island, four Wisdomkeepers appeared in a Native village. The tribe was celebrating with a feast. Everyone was happy — the children were playing, the women were visiting, the Elders were telling stories, and there was plenty of food.

Late in the evening, one of the children shouted an alarm: a canoe was approaching the river's edge. The men picked up their weapons and ran to the shore. In the canoe they saw four Elders paddling silently. They did not seem dangerous. The canoe landed gently and the men helped the Elders ashore.

The whole village rushed there to see what was happening. None of them knew who the Elders were. There were two men and two women the villagers had never seen before. Finally the oldest of them spoke: We are from a place called the Wisdomkeepers. This is the place where your ancestors live. We need to talk to your council and to your Elders.

The Elders and the villagers headed back toward the feast and word was sent ahead to prepare food for the guests. The village Elders seemed to know who the strange Elders were, even though the rest of the village had no idea. The new Elders ate in silence. Finally, Old Crow Man, the village medicine man, reached into the back of the tipi to get a very old, worn pouch. He untied it and brought out the sacred pipe. He slowly filled it, pointed it to the four directions and then laid it carefully on a cloth by the fire.

4

Members of the community waited outside the teepee until the silence was broken by the sound of the tribal drum and singers offering a welcome song. This was the custom, to sing an honor song for guests. After the song, silence fell again, broken only by the rippling water, the crackling fire, and sometimes the sound of a baby stirring.

Then the four Elders stood up and the oldest one spoke:

"My name is Standing Bear. We are from a place that is far away from here. It is called the place of the Wisdomkeepers, where all knowledge is kept, where all the secrets of the Universe are kept. We have come here to tell you about your future. And we will tell you what we want from you.

"Very soon, you will be meeting the light-skins. These people come from a great distance. Their numbers are great. When they come to your country they will do strange things. They will cut down the trees, dig minerals from the earth, they will kill your children and your women, and they will take your land. They will not live in harmony. They will be very greedy. They will not honor your culture nor will they honor your traditions. They will take your children away and teach them their own ways. They will try to make you forget your teachings.

"The People will live in a time of turmoil, difficulty, and oppression. Everything will be taken from you. The light-skins will not honor Mother Earth and her teachings. The two-legged, the four-legged, even the Eagles will almost be destroyed.

"You will be subjected to four tests called mind-changers. If you weaken and give in to the mind-changers, the People will perish and the Indian way of traditional thinking will be lost. The first test will be a liquid; the second test will be black robes with a black book; the third test will be a song, and the fourth test will be a card.

"This testing period is necessary and will cause great problems among the People. The only thing you will be allowed to keep will be your spirituality. Everything else will be taken. Your spirituality will be tested.

"The testing time will end when the sun is blocked in the seventh moon. Then the People will enter a time of harmony. During the early part of the springtime, a great healing will occur: a white buffalo calf will appear in the north. A healing wind will form in the northeast and will gain strength. When it is strong, it will blow to the south. Then it will turn and blow to the west, then to the north. This will be the path of the great healing.

"During the healing time, your medicine knowledge will return. You will see the eagles come back. You will see the buffalo come back. You will find medicine bundles. During the great healing, many people will be chosen as healers. Each of them will be given a certain talent and gift. These talents and gifts will be needed to help the people learn to live in harmony once again. Many of these people will suffer difficulties and setbacks that will prepare them for their healing journey.

"The Wisdomkeepers will start to appear to some of these healers. The Wisdomkeepers will be guiding the healing. They will appear to certain individuals and impart ancient knowledge to them. The task of those individuals is to share the teachings with the world. And so the world will heal."

Another Elder stood: "My name is Shining Star," she said. "The reason we are telling you these things is because we bring a request from the Wisdomkeepers to your village. You have the knowledge of living in harmony with the Earth. You have kept the traditional ways and are still living them. We have been observing some of your young people, Two Eagles, Two Moons, and a young woman named Morning Star. We have also been observing the Elder, Tak-na. We would like to take these four with us to the place of the Wisdomkeepers. You will not see them again. When the great healing takes place, we will put them back on the Earth among the People so they can guide the People back to the traditional knowledge. We know you need to talk these things over. We will wait tonight by the river. If you are willing for them to come with us, be there by sunrise." And they went away to the river.

Word of this conversation spread throughout the village. No one could sleep. Everyone waited for the decision of the council. Two Moons, Two Eagles, Morning Star and Tak-na were summoned to the council house. Finally the council approached the people to explain. The chief held his talking stick high in the air until the people were quiet. Then he spoke. "We have sat in council and listened to our visitors from the Wisdomkeepers. They showed us through the sacred crystals what the future of our people is going to be. We saw the turbulent times that our grandchildren will suffer. We also saw the time of healing that will come. In order for the healing to happen, it will be necessary for the people to learn again what we all know to be true today. Our traditional knowledge will be lost and our grandchildrens' children will not be aware of it any more. To insure the survival of our people, we have approved a plan to preserve our knowledge and return it to our descendants to begin the time of healing."

At sunrise, the four chosen ones went to the river to begin their journey to the place of the Wisdomkeepers.

The Eagle Called My Name

It was early spring and the warmth of the sun was putting life into every living thing. The forest was full of birds building their nests and fish flopping in the ponds and streams. All of nature was in motion to create the next generation of life. After the long, quiet winter, the village was coming alive, its people once again figuring out how to live in modern society. Since the white people came to live in Indian country, confusion had been the normal state of affairs. Where once everyone began the day with prayer and ceremony, now there were the sounds of TV and radio, as well as the presence of the Internet. Instead of teaching their children in the traditional ways, parents yelled at them, trying to get them off to school. Anxiety pervaded the community like an invisible fog.

A few of the people tried to live in the traditional way, but they were often criticized by those who had become "modern:" they gossiped, belittling and judging them. This situation caused a great frustration among the Elders. They quietly kept watch for any young person who was interested in learning the old ways.

Yesterday little Maggie turned six years old. Her grandfather watched her while her mother helped out at the tribal offices. Grandfather noticed again that she was different from the other children. As a baby, she had been unusually quiet and as a child she was prayerful. She seemed to be able to communicate with animals. Often a butterfly would light on her arm. She was attracted to flowers and smiled when one was put under her nose or brushed against her cheek. She enjoyed playing with other children, but never minded being alone. Her favorite place was by the water. Grandfather wondered how she stayed so stable. Her father drank too much and her mother was always busy trying to make ends meet. But little Maggie remained cheerful and calm.

One day she came to her grandfather. "Grandfather, can we go fishing at the Point?"

"Why, of course," said grandfather. He loved this little girl. He had been present when she was born. He had seen the blue light over her head and knew she was born for a very special purpose. Maggie's mother had watched the tears roll down his face the first time he held his grandchild. There was a spiritual bond between them. The first word Maggie said was momma, and the second was Tak-Na, Grandfather. When she was a toddler and he came by her house, she would run to him, calling Tak-Na, Tak-Na. Grandfather was always happy to be with her.

So now the two of them went off in their canoe, planning to fish during the day, camp by the water at night, and return in the morning.

Grandfather paddled the canoe and little Maggie sat in front, letting the cool ocean breeze blow in her face. She liked being with her grandfather because he made her feel so comfortable and safe. She closed her eyes, listened to the birds, smelled the salty air, and began to dream.

Soon they arrived at the Point and set up camp. Then Grandfather picked up the fishing poles and guided little Maggie down to the water. It was calm and Maggie sensed it would be a good day for fishing. By noon they had caught enough fish for dinner. Then Grandfather said he would go across the channel and asked Maggie if she would rather go with him or stay and fish. Maggie knew she would be able to see him working across the channel so she decided to stay at the camp. Grandfather took the canoe and set off toward the island.

Maggie lay on the grass gazing at the sky. She watched the seagulls floating effortlessly, making lazy eights. Sometimes she would close her eyes against the bright sun and then she would listen to her surroundings. Suddenly, she felt a shadow cross her face. She opened her eyes and sensed a form of life in the blinding sun. It felt mysterious. Soon she could see that it was a very large bird. She sat up. The bird screeched very loudly. The sound was so strange it sent a chill through her body. The bird was an Eagle. Maggie noticed it was flying toward her. It screeched again. Maggie felt it was trying to talk to her. She stood up, wishing Grandfather was there. Slowly the Eagle came closer, then folded its wings and went into a dive. As it passed over, she could feel the wind from its wings. Shivers went through her body. When the Eagle circled and called out again, Maggie distinctly heard her name. As the Eagle passed above her, a feather fell and slowly swirled down. Maggie stretched out her hands and caught the Eagle feather.

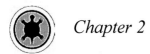 *Chapter 2*

Grandfather, What Does This Mean?

Little Maggie sat on the ground, no longer interested in fishing. Only the Eagle feather convinced her she had not been dreaming. She watched her grandfather across the channel and wanted to tell him what had happened. She could have called to him, but knew it was better to wait.

Finally she saw him loading the canoe and paddling back toward her. When he was settled in at the camp, she climbed onto his lap and told him every detail of her story. Then she asked, "Grandfather, what does this mean?"

Grandfather set her down on the ground. He took a braid of sweetgrass from his medicine bag, lit it, and smudged the Eagle feather and Maggie. He looked at her with tears in his eyes. Then he spoke.

"Maggie, I have always known you were special. I never knew why I felt this until today. In the old days, the Elders told us that when certain people were chosen by the Creator to do something special, something unique, he would send an Eagle. The Eagle would call their name and drop a feather in their hand. Maggie, what this means is that you are chosen by the Great Spirit to do something very special while you are on the Earth. The Eagle has called your name."

Be Silent, Little Girl

The next day, Grandfather and Maggie returned to the village. They had caught enough fish to distribute to the Elders. Grandfather cautioned Maggie not to tell anyone what had happened at the Point. He felt that no one in the community would understand.

He had watched the village people over many years. When he was a little boy the community was very poor, but the people were very close. The houses were nothing more than shacks with neither running water nor plumbing. Mostly the people fished in the summer and moved to inland camps in the winter. Often the winters were very cold, but everyone made it because everyone stuck together. There were ceremonies, dances, socials, and strong families to help everyone get through.

Grandfather wasn't sure just when the community started to get off track. Maybe it was during World War II or just thereafter. After the War, many of the community members drifted off to neighboring towns to take jobs. Some stayed away for a long time and others went back and forth between the reservation and the cities. Slowly, the community disintegrated. Many of the members started to drink and others started taking drugs. Eventually, the ceremonies stopped, the people stopped speaking their language, they stopped dancing, and they stopped caring for one another.

As the drinking continued, other problems started to show up. The men became angry and began beating their wives and children. That had not happened before. Parents began to hurt their children. The children stopped respecting them along with the other adults and Elders. As the drinking continued, the other problems also got worse. Soon the community members were fighting among themselves and nobody was getting along. Grandfather realized it had been like that for a long time.

Maggie's family was no exception. Her dad was an alcoholic and her mom was about as mean as anyone can get. All of

Maggie's brothers and sisters were in and out of trouble. But Maggie didn't get caught up in the difficulties, she seemed somehow to be protected.

By the time she was thirteen, she had gained a lot of respect. Her helpfulness to others was very visible in the community, even though she tried to do things in secret. She helped the Elders, she helped families that were struggling. She had kind words to say about everyone. If someone criticized a drunk, she would respond by saying something good about him.

At that time there were still a number of Elders who knew about ceremonies and the traditional culture. They did not force this knowledge on anyone, but hey were willing to share it with anyone who was willing to learn. These Elders noticed Maggie when she was by the water, alone, looking at the ocean; or when she was studying and listening to her teachers. Often they would watch as she opened her medicine bundle, pulled out the Eagle feather, lit some sweetgrass and sat there for hours.

When Maggie turned sixteen and other girls her age were getting interested in boys, she followed what was going on in the community. She was very frustrated with all the turmoil, with the fighting, with the drugs and alcohol. One day, she sat down by the water and burst into tears without really knowing why. Her grandfather had been watching her, so he strolled down to see if she needed to talk. Maggie was glad to see him, but she started crying even harder as he came closer. "Grandfather, I have never been so confused in all my life. My heart is very heavy and I don't even know why I'm crying. I'm so mixed up. Grandfather, what should I do?"

Grandfather decided it was time for one of the old wisdom stories.

"Maggie, the Elders tell us the stories about the cycle of life, from baby, to youth, then adult, and Elder. The four directions. The human grows in cycles and seasons, just like the trees and the salmon. As humans travel around the cycle of life, they go through four seasons. Each season lasts one year: one year of spring, one year of summer, one year of fall, and one year of winter. At the end of each cycle, you are four years older, so the third cycle took you to the age of 12, and the fourth cycle starts you into the teen years. During this time, your feelings and emotions and the changes in your body cause your thinking to develop so you can become a strong, balanced, spiritual woman. In the fourth cycle the Creator gives you three questions. The answers to those questions will help you know your identity.

"When the question **'Why am I?'** comes to you, you begin to seek the meaning of life. When you cannot answer this question, you will appear to be confused. You are searching for **purpose.**

"When you wonder **'Who am I?'** you begin to seek your own **identity,** to know who you are and who you are not. Just as the maple tree knows who it is and knows it is different from the pine tree, you must know who you are.

"When you consider **'Where am I going?'** you are seeking **direction.** The Creator meant us to be vision people. In our minds, we can make pictures. If we have vision, that determines the direction we will choose in our lives. When we know our purpose, identity, and direction, we will never be lost or disconnected.

"I want to help you find the answers to these questions. Then you will be free."

They took the canoe and headed out, passing the Point and landing at the island. Grandfather tied the canoe to a rock, helped Maggie out of the canoe, and started up the hill. As they walked, he said "I'm going to show you something that only a few of the Elders know. We have kept this a secret because our people are so sick. We knew there would be a time when we would need to show this to you. Please keep this a secret."

They stopped at a pile of brush. Grandfather moved it aside to reveal the opening of a cave. He took Maggie by the hand and they entered the darkness. Grandfather bent over to find a torch. When he lit it, Maggie could see a long tunnel and hear the faint dripping of water. They passed through the tunnel and came to a cave. Grandfather lit another torch that revealed a very large room.

On the far side of the cave was a pile of deer hides. Grandfather slowly moved them aside. Maggie was surprised to see that they had covered a very large drum and drumstick that appeared to be very old. Maggie's heart beat faster. "Many years ago" Grandfather said, "this was our tribal drum. It is very sacred. It has been with our people since the beginning of time. In the old days all the people respected and honored this drum. When the white man came, he told our children the drum was bad and that it was evil. He said we needed to follow the white man's ways. The people began to listen to the white man.

"The Elders in those days were very sad because the People stopped playing the drum. If there is no drum, the people have no heartbeat. When the drum stops, the People are dead. So the Elders hid the drum here. They said some day a special person would come along and understand the drum. When the drum starts beating again, the People will come alive and the healing will begin.

"Maggie, you are that special person who will understand about the drum and what it will do for the People. You are welcome to come to this cave anytime you want, but understand that only you can come here. Let this drum be your teacher. It will help you learn the answers to the three questions."

"But Grandfather, how will I learn this? What am I supposed to do?"

Grandfather looked at her with tears in his eyes. "Inside of every person is the knowledge of what it takes to be a good human being. The Creator wrote this knowledge in our hearts. We find this Wisdom inside of ourselves by being quiet, by being still. So be still, little girl. Come sit with the drum and be still."

14

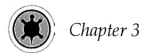 *Chapter 3*

The First Teacher

They left the cave, carefully covering the opening. That night, Maggie tossed and turned as she heard the ancestors singing. She seemed to understand the songs even though she didn't know them. The sound of the drum made her cry. She would doze off and then awake in tears as the Eagle screeched her name for the first time since she had received its feather.

She went to see Grandfather in the morning. He was about to leave for two weeks, but said she needed to spend time with the drum. The next afternoon, she took the canoe to the Island. She moved the brush aside from the cave entrance and carefully worked her way down the passage to the cavern. She uncovered the drum, offered tobacco to the four directions, and prayed. When she picked up the drumstick, it felt like magic. Maggie became very still.

She sat there for a long time until she felt a presence in the cave. Maggie spun around and saw two Elders, a man and a woman, watching her. Before she could react, the woman smiled and said, "We are friends of your grandfather. We are here to teach you the drum and the old songs. We have been waiting for you." Their smiles were so pleasant that Maggie's fear vanished.

For the rest of that day and many days afterward, Maggie was instructed by the two Elders. The more she played the drum and sang the songs, the more she felt herself becoming part of them.

Early one morning she was awakened by her grandfather, who had returned the night before. As he cooked breakfast, she told him about the Elders in the cave and asked why he hadn't told her about his friends. First, he was silent, his mouth open. Then he said they had appeared to him in a dream, holding a drum painted with a white buffalo calf. He had a hard time holding back the tears because he knew Maggie was beginning a journey of healing for the People.

After breakfast, Maggie and her grandfather strolled through the village. They came upon a group of Elders who were talking about how something different had been going on in the past few weeks. People were more friendly, people who wouldn't ordinarily speak to one another were making conversation. They said it's almost like we're coming alive. As Maggie and Grandfather walked away they had the same thought: When the people have a drum they have a heartbeat. If the people have no drum, the people are dead. The drum represents the heartbeat of the Mother Earth. The drum keeps a heart beating among the people

Maggie continued to go to the cave and learn from the Elders. They taught her songs and dances and much of the traditional culture. One day they said there would be another guest, so Maggie made sure she had her sweetgrass and tobacco to offer to the new Elder. She was called Shining Star and Maggie thought she was really special. Even among the Wisdomkeepers, there are revered Elders. Shining Star had the respect of these Elders. She carried her medicine bundle carefully attached to her side. Her hair was long and gray, her skin was wrinkled, but her eyes radiated love and caring. It was easy to see just how insightful she was. Maggie felt that Shining Star's eyes could look into her soul.

Shining Star was both serious and humorous. Maggie enjoyed her and looked forward to her visits. One day Shining Star asked Maggie to do something special, saying, "I want you to do this for me and ask no questions. Go into the forest by Willow Creek. Nearby you will see ten birch trees. Cut a wide strip of bark from each tree. Roll the strips up and tie them with leather thongs. Then bring them to me."

It took Maggie three days to carry out Shining Star's instructions. She went to Willow Creek, found the trees, and made the scrolls. She brought the scrolls to Shining Star, and was told to come back with her grandfather at the next full moon.

The Full Moon Meeting

As Grandfather and Maggie approached the hidden cave, they noticed how beautiful the moon was. They were full of anticipation. Inside, they were met not only by Shining Star but also by three other Elders.

The oldest one introduced himself. "My name is Gray Hawk. Many moons ago, we came to a village where the people knew how to live in harmony. They were happy and satisfied. The leadership of the people was done in a good way. This village had all the traditional knowledge. The Elders were respected and they taught the youth. The village was very aware of the ceremonies. All of life was a ceremony. The people had learned the lessons of nature. They knew all things had life. Plants were called the plant nation, certain animals were called the two-legged, and the four-legged. Because they lived at night, the stars were called the star nation. All living things were considered relations. The people showed tremendous respect for all living things."

Maggie's heart beat fast and cold sweat started to run down her body. She felt lonely and abandoned. The Elder's words were familiar, but she didn't understand why. Grandfather, too, was disturbed. The Elder's conversation brought up lost memories and feelings he had never experienced before. He stared at the ground tearfully, feeling heavy-hearted. When he reached over and touched Maggie's hand, he felt her shaking.

The fire was warm but seemed to make the night more mysterious. Maggie and Grandfather sat silently, each afraid to ask the questions that might explain their new-found feelings.

Gray Hawk continued. "I suppose both of you are wondering who we are. It's time we tell you. There are other worlds along with the one you live in. We are from one of those worlds. It is called the place of the Wisdomkeepers. There are 40 Elders who are allowed to be there. Our job is to guard the wisdom. We can live in either the physical world or the spiritual world. We can come and go as we please. You will only remember this conversation when you are here in the cave. When you leave the cave, you will not remember that we told you who we are. This is for your protection as well as ours."

"You were both taken from the old village, many moons ago, and kept in the place of the Wisdomkeepers because we knew the white man was coming to Turtle Island and we knew he would destroy everything he touched. We knew he would even destroy Mother Earth. We knew his ways were not the way of spirit and harmony but the ways of destruction and greed. We had to hide the wisdom because it would be needed to turn the destruction around. You were taken from the old village to be returned during the time of healing. This information also, you will only remember while you are in this cave. When you leave the cave, you will not remember your true identity."

Shining Star made some tea and poured a powder into it. As Maggie and Grandfather drank it, they began to remember the village. They began to remember their friends. They began to remember the night the Old Ones came to the village. Maggie began to remember her life as Two Moons. She remembered Two Eagles and how they were to be married the summer that the Elders came. She remembered the painful departure from Two Eagles. She remembered their last night together, cuddled by the water's edge when they both knew the journey had to be taken. They had been taught that decisions must always be for the People and that sacrifice is spiritual. Each of them had been taught to put themselves last and the People first. If they were to make a decision, the main question was whether it would be of benefit for all the people. The power of sacrifice comes when you decide to put yourself last. Because we are all interconnected, all small parts of something bigger, the individual sometimes sacrifices itself for the good of the whole. In order to survive, the people must come first.

Maggie broke out in loud sobs, glanced at Grandfather and then fell on her knees in front of the Wisdomkeepers. She cried out, "Two Eagles was also taken by the Old Ones, is he here too? Will I be able to see him again?" Shining Star walked over to her and with a gentle, wrinkled hand raised Maggie's head and looked in her eyes with great kindness. "Two Eagles is also on the Earth in another community a great distance from here. But yes, you will meet again at a gathering of the Elders. At first you won't recognize each other, but you will meet, you will get married in a traditional way, and your lives will be spent in healing many Indian communities. But, my child, when you leave here, you won't remember this."

Slowly the sadness left Maggie's heart as feelings of love, security and understanding came to her. Now she understood why she had no interest in the young men who approached her. Her heart was already committed to Two Eagles.

Grandfather listened and watched and for the first time in his life felt at peace.

Now Gray Hawk sat down and another Elder, Looking Cloud, stood up to speak.

"When the white man came, he brought his ways and taught them to the Indian people, saying they would be good for us. So the Indian people went that way, but it was not a good road, it was a road of destruction. On this road there were alcohol, drugs, family breakups, loss of culture, loss of spirituality. Living this new way caused the people and the leadership to lose the spiritual way of life; thus disharmony became their way of life.

"Now the Indian nations are in a time when great healing is going to occur. There are going to be many changes. In order for these changes to happen, the Native leadership must change. The white man's system of leadership will not work in Indian communities. The white man's system is very outwardly oriented. He is very selfish and seeks power and control. He says it is not right to mix God and work. He says spirituality is separate. He has built a place where he goes to worship one day a week. He has designed a system that uses guilt, shame, and fear to control people. If you simply make a mistake, you are made to feel that there is something wrong with you. His greatest error is his disrespect for women. He does not respect women as being intelligent and having value.

"He is so greedy that he will ignore his family and the responsibility of teaching his children. It has gotten so bad that his children are killing each other. The white man doesn't respect the Earth. He thinks he can do anything to Her, he thinks he can put poison in Her waters, he thinks he can cut down all the trees, he thinks the Earth is here to serve him. He treats the Earth just as he treats his women. He thinks he can do this and escape the consequences. He has no knowledge of interconnectedness. He thinks only of separation.

"We Indian people are doing this too, but the difference is that we know better because it is written in our hearts that everything is connected. We know what we do because the knowledge is handed down from our ancestors within. Inside each person are the ancestors. All of your grandfathers and grandmothers are with you, all the way back to the beginning of time. Their knowledge remains within.

"The prophecies say that Native people are to become the teachers of the Earth. So we need to remember our old ways, because we cannot give away what we don't have. The traditional Indian way of looking at spirituality was taught by Mother Earth. As the Elders observed nature, they learned about cycles, seasons, balance, the Seen world and the Unseen world. They learned everything was interconnected. They realized that everything contained a life force. They learned that man was to honor this interconnected system because we do not own the Earth, the Earth owns us. They learned that if we feel disharmony, we must look within ourselves because that is where the disharmony exists. All things must be treated with honor and respect because the life force of the Creator is in all things.

"We Elders from the place of the Wisdomkeepers are doing spiritual intervention on the Earth. The Earth is headed for a big conflict. The powers that are in place are collapsing. The leadership, the governments are corrupt. They are spiritually sick. They are more concerned with the gross national product than the gross national spirit. So the Elders are bringing back knowledge about the old traditional ways and the first lesson is about leadership.

"Inside of every person is the traditional knowledge that we call the ancestors within. When the ancestors within hear the truth, or values, or principles and laws, they wake you up and tell you to pay attention. The teachings are written inside every human being."

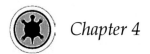 *Chapter 4*

The Scrolls For Leadership

"Maggie, we had you gather ten pieces of birch bark. We took the scrolls to the place of the Wisdomkeepers and recorded the ancient knowledge about leadership on them. Each scroll has a symbol. When the ancestors inside you see one of these symbols, they will wake up and whisper one of the secrets of leadership to you.

"Sit here," Shining Star said, gesturing toward a buffalo robe that was spread by the fire. "Close your eyes." The penetrating odor of cedar smoke came to Maggie. Then she felt its medicine engulfing her body. The voice of another Elder began an old song. Maggie felt herself settling into a very quiet place within.

She heard someone unrolling a scroll, but remained still until she was told to open her eyes slowly. Across the crackling fire the Elder held the scroll. Maggie saw the symbol on it and felt a stirring near her heart. She closed her eyes and heard a clear, gentle voice within. The voice resonated, not only in her mind, but throughout every cell of her body.

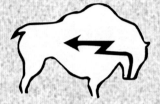

Scroll One

Change Is From Within

The arrow pointing from the mouth to the heart means that all solutions and answers are written within. If you look to your heart before you speak, you can only speak the truth. Inside of every salmon is the innate knowledge of what it takes to be a good salmon. Inside of every deer is the innate knowledge of what it takes to be a good deer. Inside of every tree is the innate knowledge of what it takes to be a good tree. It causes an oak tree to be an oak and a pine tree to be a pine. We human beings have not been left out. Inside of every human being is the innate knowledge of its own wellbeing, knowledge of how to develop oneself emotionally, mentally, physically and spiritually. This knowledge is the key to the development of a leader. You must not depend on what the white man has taught you, but instead

on the knowledge of what the Creator wrote in
your heart. The leaders of the old communities
held an Eagle feather or the Sacred Pipe over
their hearts to show that they were speaking with a
good mind and a good spirit. The heart is where
the ancient knowledge was hidden. That is where
you must look, if you are really dedicated to
leading our Native people from sickness into
healing. There is the knowledge of how to
become a servant leader.

The first secret you must know is this: Repeated
thinking about something will create a habit.
Once you have the habit of thinking about
something, then you will automatically think
according to the pattern of thought. If you have
created a habit of negative thinking, then you will
automatically think negatively. If you have
created a pattern of blaming others, you will do
that automatically. It stays this way until you
replace the old thought pattern with a new one.
Only a habit can change a habit. Habits are
changed by using repetition. Repetition is the
mother of change. If you want to change your

life, change your thinking. Repeat this teaching to yourself four times a day, from one full moon to the next:

Today, I will practice changing myself, for I know I can't change anyone else. Each morning as I prepare to lead the community, I will remember that my real power is in knowing I can change myself.

The second secret is:
I must be the change I wish to see in the community.

If I want to see respect in the community, then I must first become respectful. I cannot give away something I don't have.

I must be the change I wish to see in the community.

If I get irritated at someone or something, I will realize it's not because of what's going on, but how I'm looking at what's going on. To find the point of view I need, I will practice looking inside for the innate knowledge. There are two viewpoints to everything; the viewpoint of the Mouse and the viewpoint of the Eagle. The Eagle and the Mouse see things differently. Today I will see that other people also have valid views.

Today if I become irritated or doubtful, I will change my viewpoint by looking inside myself.

I must be the change I wish to see in the community.

Each morning I will plan the development of my character. I will look inside myself for the knowledge of what I can become. I will develop my being and voice my intent. I will pray, saying, "My Creator, you have chosen me to lead my people. Today, I need your help. Left on my own, I will struggle, but with the guidance of the spiritual world, I will grow and develop myself into a leader for the future. With the Creator's help, I can develop into a spiritual leader. Oh Great Spirit, teach me to change myself. Give me the tools to look within because that is where the answers are.

You have written inside me all the leadership principles I need to know. Today, if I become stubborn or angry, teach me to pause before I speak, for my words have power, like throwing a spear. My words can hurt people or my words can heal people. Today I ask you to direct my thinking. If I become confused, let me look within, to the place where you wait for me to come to you for advice."

I must be the change I wish to see in the community.

The only way I can lead my community back to wellness is if I am well myself. I cannot give away what I don't have. Today I make myself available to change. I want to be an effective leader. I choose to ask for your help.

I must be the change I wish to see in the community.

Only as I change myself can I develop as an effective leader of Indian people.

My future is in your hands.
I humbly ask for your help!

The Elder rolled up the scroll and tied it with the thong. Maggie was beginning to understand. She had been trained to believe the ancient knowledge was lost, but the wisdom had been inside all along. She had forgotten to look inside. The Elder reached behind a rock and pulled out the second scroll. Maggie opened her eyes, took in the new symbol, then closed her eyes and opened to the inner voice.

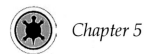 *Chapter 5*

Scroll Two

Use the Powers of the East

The voice spoke again: During the second moon, you need to say this four times a day until the cycle is complete...

Scroll Two

Use the Powers of the East
The Direction of New Energy

I will use the powers of the East each morning. I will rise early to access the power, for this is the best time. These are the powers that start the birds singing. These are the powers that wake up the flowers. This is the direction from which flows new energy. This direction holds the powers of creativity. As I face the East and feel the sun rise up, it gives me the gifts of freshness, energy and creativity. I will close my eyes and focus on my blessings. Today, I can see. Today, I can hear. Today, I can smell, I can walk. Today I intend to be happy. Today I will have peace of mind. Today I will sing. Today is my day for lessons. Today I will live as if it is my last day. Today I will live in the present, I will not cloud my mind with future thoughts. I will rid my mind of any thoughts of the past. Today is the only time that changes can be made. I cannot change the future, nor can I alter the past.

I look forward with great expectations. This morning I take the hand of the Creator and walk through the day with confidence, for I know the Creator is with me. This morning I ask the Creator to guide my thinking and remove from me any dishonesty, self-pity, and self-seeking motives. Today I am proud to be Indian. I walk in leadership like the ancestors. I am a good leader because of my relationship with the Great Spirit.

This is what my ancestors did. They got up early each morning to greet the day and receive the powers from the sun. They set their intent and sent out morning thoughts for all the people. They prayed for their community. They considered it an honor to serve the people. This will become my habit. I will practice this today and every day until I do it naturally.

I love my people.

The Elder turned to Maggie and said, "Here is another secret of the ancient leaders.

"The morning window of power exists only from when the sun first starts to rise until you can see the whole circle of the sun. When this window is open the powers are transferred. If you wait until the sun is higher in the sky, you have missed the window. This is the only time it is available. It is good to offer tobacco or to burn sage or sweetgrass. This is the time to be blessed by special powers."

Maggie opened her eyes. The fire cast shadows of the Elders present. She felt as if she was experiencing history in the making. At moments she wondered, what is really going on here? Why am I involved in such a sacred happening? Of all the people who could have been chosen, why me? She sat on the buffalo robe, in silence, pondering. She heard the unrolling of another scroll and wondered what the next symbol would be.

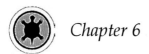 *Chapter 6*

Scroll Three

Use the Powers of the South

Slowly, the Elder turned the scroll so Maggie could see it in the light of the fire. "Oh," she thought, "the sun at midday." She closed her eyes and once again felt the interconnectedness in her body as the inner voice returned...

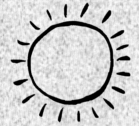

Scroll Three

Use the Powers of the South
The Direction of the Sun

The South holds the powers for use during the day. During the time of the third moon, saying this four times a day will add to the power that the ancient ones knew. Remember, repetition is the mother of change. Say this to yourself:

As I proceed through the day, I will encounter setbacks, conflicts, problems, and challenges. As a leader I need to understand these conflicts are my friends. They are my keys to growth. During the day, all of nature is going through conflict. If a seed is planted in the ground, the shell of the seed is trying to crack open and the white young roots are fighting their way through the soil. The stem is struggling to get to the surface of the earth. Eventually, with the power of persistence, the stem breaks through the soil. So it is through a system of conflict that this seed becomes a blooming flower. The natural law says that for anything to grow it must first struggle to do so. Inside of every conflict is the solution. Conflict precedes clarity. My new way is to make the conflict my friend. Today I will embrace the conflict because it is my friend. I know the solution is inside the conflict. As a good leader I will attract the conflict, for that is what leaders do. We solve and resolve conflict. I will also make every setback my friend, for I know every setback is only temporary. I will develop tenacity. If I encounter a setback, I will go around it, through it, over it, or under it. I need this attitude in order to lead the people.

The powers of the South will help me do this. The Creator is always with me. I can call on his power and wisdom. Today I will be a spiritual thinker. Today I will practice and develop the thinking skills of my ancestors. They chose to be spiritual leaders, therefore I will use the same powers to develop myself. I will use the powers of the south. Today I am a positive thinker. I will create in myself a good mind. When I am presented with conflict, I will look inside before I speak. I will realize conflict is my guidance system. I need this input to lead my people to wellness.

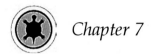 *Chapter 7*

Scroll Four

Use the Powers of the West

Scroll Four

Use the Powers of the West
The Direction of Letting Go

The direction of the West is where the sun sets. This is the direction of letting go, the direction of forgiveness and the direction of examining how the day went. Each evening I have the choice of being free. In order to be a servant leader, I must be free of resentments. Resentment is poison to my very soul. Carrying resentment against another person is like taking poison and hoping the other person will die. Resentment blocks the powers of the Creator.

I realize I must forgive, even the unforgivable. And I especially need to forgive myself.

I cannot be a servant leader if I am full of resentment. Therefore, each evening I will examine myself: Did I hold any resentments today? Was I selfish today? Was I dishonest or deceitful? Did I act or react from fear? Was I thinking about the people first? Was I kind and considerate to all? Do I owe anyone an apology?

I will consider these questions and answer them so I don't have any blockage to the power. After I think about the day, if I do owe someone an apology, I will contact them immediately and let them know I was wrong. When I do this evening review, I will face the West because this is the direction of letting go. Just as the sun sets, the world around me starts to shut down. The birds tuck their heads under their wings, the wind quiets down and the eagle returns to its nest. This is the time to clear my mind of what happened today. Now it is past.

Also, I will review what I did right today. I will remember the times of confusion and how I secretly asked the Creator for guidance. In this way, I will prepare my mind for a peaceful rest. I will allow the powers of the west to draw what is negative from my mind and return it to peace. I pray that the Creator will forgive my wrongs and that while I sleep, He will feed my mind the corrections I need to make. Then I will start the next day as a better leader.

I will look at the bigger picture. I will realize many of my people have been wounded by alcohol and abuse. If I'm attacked, I won't take it personally. I know attacks are not so much about me, but more about someone's unresolved issues – something that happened when they were a child, or a hurt that never healed. When people need love most is when they deserve it least. I will practice being loving.

I will use these spiritual tools until they become natural parts of my being. Each night, I will be free from things I missed during the day. If I carry my own hurts day after day, I will lose my effectiveness. I will keep my mind clear just as my ancestors did. Each night I will let go and be free. Each night I will fall asleep in the arms of the Creator.

As the voice continued to reveal the ancient teachings, Maggie felt very moved. She saw that hope could come to her community, like water for a wilting plant. She sensed that the teachings would bring about a permanent change that would overcome the devastations of alcohol, drugs, and violence so the community could begin to heal.

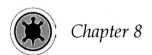 *Chapter 8*

Scroll Five

Use the Powers of the North

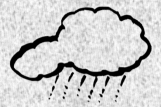

Scroll Five

Use the Powers of the North
The Direction of Wisdom

Today I call on the powers of the North. This is the direction of the Elders and the source of wisdom. Just because I am called a leader doesn't mean I always know the way. No person can grow without the help of other people and the help of the Elders. When I feel weak or lost, I will face the North and pray for wisdom. When I feel afraid, I will pray to the North and ask for wisdom. When I feel alone, I will face the North and ask for guidance. The spirits send their powers from the North.

It is said that the person who has wisdom, has everything. By praying to the North each day, I will grow in wisdom so as to help the people. Today, I make it my goal to be a wise leader just like my ancestors. The ancestors who were effective leaders always became so with prayer. Today, I will learn to depend on the Creator as my advisor. By doing this, my decision and insight will be good and fair. I will practice getting the wisdom from the North.

The Elders say pray to the four directions. They say there are powers that will come and help us. From the four directions, I will receive the spiritual tools of the old ways. To the north I will say, "I come before you a humble person, realizing I know nothing. I come before you in a pitiful way. My head, without my heart, is my enemy. I need your strength and wisdom. I need your power to direct my thinking. Make me strong so I can face my people without shame. Let me stand before you, open to receive the wisdom.

Maggie heard an Elder singing softly. She smelled the strong aroma of cedar and watched its smoke swirling upward. There was a sense of change and hope in the air. Maggie felt the ancient teachings coming to life again. They had not disappeared, they were only forgotten.

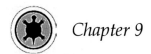 *Chapter 9*

Scroll Six

Interconnectedness

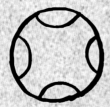

Scroll Six

Interconnectedness
We Are All Related

Today, I will remember we are all interconnected. I will remember that even though I have the title of leader, I am of the same worth as everyone else. Everything on the Mother Earth is connected. The Earth is my mother. All the two-leggeds are my relations. The sun is my father. Every community member is my relative. Every Indian child is my child. Every Indian woman is my sister. Every Indian man is my brother. I will remember this, too, so I treat each one as a relative. They are important. If they are unemployed, I will listen. If they have problems with alcohol, I will listen. If I'm approached by a single parent, I will listen. If the one talking to me is a teenager, I will listen, for this is my child. Today, I will not ignore anyone. Whenever they speak to me, I will give them my full attention. I will think of how we are connected. This is the way of my ancestors. I will remember that the pain of one is the pain off all, and the honor of one is the honor of all. When I sit in a meeting and hear about problems, I will think of my connectedness to the whole community.

The white man has taught us to think in boxes, lines of separation and division. I will take the organization chart as it is today, turn it upside down and put the people on top and the leadership on the bottom. I will not pay attention to the boxes and the lines of separation in the organization chart. I will realize that in the spiritual way, everything is interconnected. I will remember that every choice or decision I make has an effect on everyone. Now I will think in circles and remember the invisible webs that connect everything. I will remember everything is alive. I will look at our schools, mental health agencies, tribal administrations, churches, youth groups, Elders and other agencies as being interconnected. Instead of using power and control, I will lead by service. I will think interconnectedness. Nature is interconnected. Communities are interconnected. Today I will see interconnectedness in all things. As an Indian leader, I will recognize our interconnectedness: that is where our power lives.

More cedar was added to the fire. The voice continued to share the teachings. It seemed it was saying something everybody already knew, but had just forgotten. There is a saying that our ancestors live inside of every human being. When we hear teachings, the ancestors inside wake up. This waking up makes us feel connected to teachings and we feel as if we knew it all along.

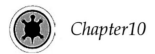 *Chapter10*

Scroll Seven

The Power of Spirituality

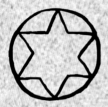

Scroll Seven

The Power of Spirituality

First, if I am to be spiritual, I must be sober. My body must be free of mind-changers. Every culture is given a gift and every gift has an enemy. The gift given to Indian people is spirituality and the enemy of spirituality is alcohol. Even one drink has an affect on the gift. People of other cultures seem to be able to drink and it has no affect on them. They can drink because they have different gifts and different enemies. The Indian people are not allowed to drink. Our gift, which will help the world, is our spirituality. Therefore, we must sacrifice the drink.

My effectiveness as a leader in my community is related to my spiritual development. Therefore, I need to understand the power of prayer. Every meeting will begin with prayer.

The most important thing I can do during the course of the day is to begin it with prayer. We are spiritual people. We have access to spiritual laws and spiritual values. These are the only weapons that will save Indian communities. We need to restore the traditional ways and do ceremonies, so I will learn the ceremonies myself. We need to dance, so I will learn the dances myself. We need to sing the old songs, so I will learn them myself. I will respect my own spirituality and will not judge the spirituality of others. All paths lead to the Creator. When the young people see me doing these things they will recognize the good ways and take them up. I will lead by example.

The next symbol appeared in the light. The inner voice continued.

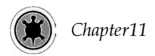 *Chapter11*

Scroll Eight

Decisions Are For the People First

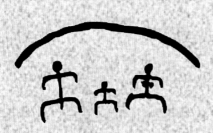

Scroll Eight

Decisions Are For the People First

Decisions are made for the good of the people first, for the good of the clan second, for the good of the family third, and for the good of self, fourth. A servant leader puts the people ahead of him or herself. The people or nation are the first priority. The ancient leaders' consideration was for the people first. They did not lead by bossing people around, controlling, or using power over them. They led by service. They were there to serve the people. When a decision was to be made, they gathered the people and discussed the situation. They did not make decisions that would best serve their clan or family. Decisions were made for the good of the whole tribe. The communities were interdependent. The leaders did not make decisions to benefit themselves. They made decisions for the good of the community.

As a leader of Indian people, I too will make decisions for the good of the tribe. I will select the best qualified members for tribal jobs. I will select the best leaders, who will also make decisions for the good of the community. I will listen to all the people and make decisions that will benefit everyone. If I get confused, I will pray to the Great Spirit for guidance.

Oh Great Spirit, help me to see the best way to decide so that the whole community will benefit. Let me not be influenced by selfish or self-seeking motives. Help me to make good choices and decisions for the people first.

The ancestors who were leaders never had an organizational chart the way corporations and organizations today do. They didn't know about top-down decision making. Their leadership always put the needs of the People first.

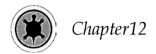 *Chapter12*

Scroll Nine

Conflict Precedes Clarity

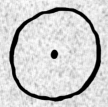

Scroll Nine

Conflict Precedes Clarity

When the Creator made the universe, he left it to be run by a set of principles, laws and values. The mother Earth is governed by those same principles, laws and values. If we live in harmony with those laws, there are certain results that will occur. If we live out of harmony, the natural laws will let us experience the consequences.

Today, I will learn that conflict is the friend of the servant leader. Conflict is what will guide me as the leader. When people complain, I will realize they are really telling me something is out of harmony. The natural laws are about harmony. Inside the seed of conflict is the harmony that I seek to solve the problem. I will not avoid conflict, I will embrace it for the solution is within it.

The natural laws say that when anything grows or changes, it must go through conflict to do so. During times of conflict, I will be the one who is calm.

The Circle defines harmony. Surrounding the Circle is a field of conflict. As long as the Circle stays a Circle there is harmony. If any part of the circle goes out of harmony, it triggers conflict. Conflict will trigger our emotions as some form of stress, anxiety or tension. This will be my secret to recognize conflict as a friend. When conflict occurs, I will use the powers of the four directions to help me find the answer.

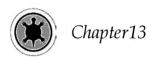 *Chapter13*

Scroll Ten
Use the Values Given By Mother Earth

Respect

Honesty

Integrity

Commitment

Understanding

Trust

Love

Communication

Scroll Ten

Use the Values Given By Mother Earth

The source of values is Mother Earth. Love is at the center of the circle and the lines show the values that are aligned with love. These are the values that Indian leadership should use. This symbol shows how values connect us to the Earth. By living the values we will establish harmony on the Earth and harmony in our communities. That is why it's important to be a value-based leader. Living the values that are given by the Earth will also allow us to become effective in our relationships. The core values of the Earth are *respect, honesty, integrity, commitment, understanding, trust, love,* and *communication.*

I will develop a code to guide my life and help me through conflicts. I will build all my relationships upon this code. When I conduct meetings I will state this code at the beginning. I will be known for living by this code. I will develop myself so strongly that I won't have to tell anyone I am doing this, for the people will know by my actions. I will pray each morning for the Great Spirit to give me knowledge of this way of life so I can live by the values of Mother Earth.

RESPECT

I am respectful to all my relations. I realize everyone has a point of view. It's by differences that we are strong. I will honor those differences. I realize that every circle has an East, a West, a North and a South. Each point on the circle has an opposite; that is what makes the circle strong. I will respect myself, both my strengths and my weaknesses, for through my weaknesses I learn the lessons of wisdom and the knowledge of the Great Spirit. My weakness will cause conflict, and inside this conflict is the truth that I seek. My faults are my friends, not my enemies. I will accept my weaknesses for they are also God's gift. The natural way to learn is through trial and error. This is how I will improve.

I will respect Mother Earth, for She is the source of life. I will watch Her, for Her knowledge is greater than any book I can read. I only need to spend time with Her and watch and listen. She is the greatest teacher. When I am troubled, I will go and sit in the woods, by the water, in the desert, in the mountains. These are the places I will go to learn.

In order to be respected, I must first be respectful.

HONESTY

A leader who is honest will always attract respect from others. It's only when I feel fear that I will be dishonest. All fear fits in two categories: either I'm going to lose something I have, or I won't get something I want. I need to remember the Creator owns everything. The things I have are only given to me to take care of. Today, I will be honest. In this way, I will be able to look with straight eyes and I will hold my head up with honor. I will not have hidden agendas and I will play no more games.

INTEGRITY

I will strive for balance as a servant leader so I will be known as a person of good character in all that I do. My reputation serves the People. I'll cultivate consistency and truthfulness in my dealings with individuals, the community, and with the diverse communities I deal with in our tribe's or organization's name. Although leadership responsibilities can be demanding, I will place reliability and keeping promises high on my list of priorities. To have integrity means to be whole. I will be known as a Native man or woman of honor in my personal life as well as in leadership.

COMMITMENT

My word is good. If I say it, you can count on it. I will watch my commitments so I stay in balance. I am of no use to the people if I am out of balance. I will be a leader whose word is good. I will pay attention to the little things, for it is by making my word good in little things that I will develop my new habits. People like to work with leaders who pay attention to the little things. I will say what I will do and I will do what I say I will do. This was the reputation of my ancestors and this will be the reputation I will have.

My words will also be good for me. I will eliminate *shoulda, coulda, woulda,* from my vocabulary. I will not be a wisher. I will not spend my mental energy wishing. If I catch myself doing so, I will halt this conversation, and ask myself, how good is your word? Are you saying things to yourself that are wasting energy? Today, I will make my word good to myself. If I say it to myself then I will act on it.

UNDERSTANDING

The Old Ones say, think like a Circle. Every Circle has an East-West-North-South. People who are standing in the East will not see the same thing as the people who are standing in the West. People who are standing in the North will not see the same thing as people who are standing in the South. People see things and feel things differently. To appreciate this, I need to have understanding. This doesn't mean I nod my head, it means that I really understand. I need to place myself in their part of the Circle to see it as they do. If an Elder explains something to me, I need to see it from an Elder's point of view. If a youth explains something to me, I need to see it from the youth's point of view. If a mom explains something to me, I need to see it from her point of view. If I do this, I will gain understanding. When I understand, I will gain respect and trust. I will be an understanding leader. This value will help me be an effective leader.

TRUST

Of all the values I can develop within myself, trust will give me the greatest advantage. I will be someone the people can trust. How do I do this? When I am with people, I will be attentive to them. When they are speaking, I will not let my mind be somewhere else. I will realize they are my relatives. I will not gossip about them or repeat something they told me in confidence. When I give my word, I will keep it. Sometimes I will need to tell them something they don't want to hear, but I will speak truthfully. I will make my commitments good. If I say I will be there, I will not only be there, but I will be there on time. Each morning I will pray to the Creator to help me develop myself in the area of trust. Leadership is based on trust.

LOVE

The power behind all values is love. Respect, commitment, honesty and trust are just other names for love. If I have love within myself, I will see love when I look at others. If I have hate inside myself, I will see hate when I look at others. It is said, love thy neighbor as thyself, and that's the problem, most of us do. I not only need to love others but I need to love myself. Love is a decision. Love is a law. Love is. Love isn't something I can give away or get. It's a power that I need to use. The love force is already there. Like gravity, it's already there, I just need to use it. I need to become a loving leader.

COMMUNICATION

The greatest orators in the world are the Native people. Our ancestors were known for their ability to speak. Many of the greatest speeches in the world have been delivered by Native people. The reason for this is our gift of spirituality. Our words may not be proper English, but the spirit behind our words makes up for it. We see with the eye of the heart. We speak from the heart. When we talk to our own people, we must use this natural gift. We must speak the truth, for only the truth can make us free. This was the way of the ancestors, and this will be my way from now on. I will be a great speaker because I speak from the principles. I will speak from the heart and see from the eye of the heart. This is how I will speak to my people.

The fire in the cave flickered as the Elders wrapped up the last scroll. Maggie and Grandfather sat in silence, wondering what would happen next. Another log was put on the fire and the cave became bright again. An Elder took a ball of sage and set it close to the fire. Slowly the heat from the fire ignited the sage and its smoke began spiraling up, taking the medicine to the spirit world. Shining Star picked up two Eagle fans, slowly lifting them up to the sky. Softly, she started to sing. The other Elders rose to their feet and joined in the song of thanks. Shining Star sang with tears rolling down her cheeks.

When the song was finished, she gave the scrolls to Maggie.

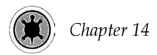 *Chapter 14*

Reunion

"These scrolls must be made known to the leaders," Shining Star said. "These are the instructions that go along with the scrolls."

"Each scroll must be read four times a day for one complete moon. It is best to start on the full moon. The first reading should be done early in the morning. Do the second reading when the sun is at its highest, midday. The third reading should be in the evening and the fourth just before bedtime. The morning reading should be done aloud and the next three in silence. So the first scroll is to be read during the first month, four times each day; then the second scroll should be read in the same way during the second month, and so on." Then Maggie was beckoned to the fire for a blessing. Eagle feathers were held over her as the Elders prayed. Chills ran through her body.

When Maggie and grandfather left the cave, the morning sun was just peeking over the horizon. They stood in silence as the doors of the east opened and cast the blessings of the easterly powers on them.

In the canoe they kept silent, listening to the cries of gulls and the soft sound of their paddles stroking the water. Maggie held the medicine bags in which the scrolls had been placed. Hardly able to believe what was taking place in her life, she pondered each event to make sure she would remember every detail. She was aware that she could only remember the events surrounding the scrolls.

They reached the village and headed for their homes, looking forward to some rest after the long night. As Maggie approached her home, she heard a loud screech from above. Four Eagles were circling in the sky. She understood they were calling her name. Finally, they flew off to the north, the place of the Elders.

Maggie slept through the day and night. Early the next morning, she stepped outside just as the sun was rising again. She got some tobacco and offered a morning gift to the powers of the east. She heard the birds waking. Maggie watched as the whole Earth came alive, responding to the powers of the east; she thanked the Great Spirit for the beautiful day and said a prayer for the people.

After breakfast Maggie looked at the scrolls in their medicine bags and wondered how she could fulfill the task set for her by the Elders. She felt restlessness in her heart, a stirring inside. Pacing the floor, she felt called to the cave. She phoned her grandfather but there was no answer. After more pacing, she decided to go by herself.

Even before she reached the cave, she heard the Elders drumming and singing the old songs and her heart filled with joy. The Elders noticed her and acknowledged her, but kept right on singing. When the song was finished, Shining Star, beaming with pride, offered Maggie some tea. Shining Star brushed Maggie's hair aside and looked into her eyes. Then she began to speak.

"Very soon there will be a blocking of the sun. This is a sign that a great healing process is going to begin on the Earth. Seven days after the blocking of the sun, there will be a gathering of many Elders. These Elders will be from many tribes, from the north, east, south, and west. You are to go to this gathering. Your grandfather will go with you. This gathering will last for four days. There is no need for you to ask any questions, all the arrangements are being made." Maggie had learned to trust the Elders. She finished her tea and returned to the canoe.

At her house she found a note that the chief wanted to see her. When she found him at the tribal offices, he explained that he had been invited to a gathering of Elders in Colorado. He had been planning to go but a family emergency had come up. He wanted to know if she would go in his place and represent the tribe. Maggie smiled inside and replied that she would be honored. As she turned to leave, the chief said, "Oh, by the way, your grandfather is going too." Maggie just kept smiling.

The Colorado Gathering Of Elders

When they arrived at the gathering, the sun was just setting behind the mountains. Many of the Elders had already arrived and more were on the way. A total of 40 were to be there. The resort was very rustic, like an old ranch. Nearby was a river of fast-moving water. Trout and bugs were busily teasing each other on its surface.

Tables had been set out with plenty of food. People were visiting and renewing old acquaintances. The Elders seemed happy and excitement filled the air.

After supper, Maggie felt drawn to the river. She could hear a waterfall just downstream. She got her hand drum and went to sit by the falls. She wanted to think. The moon's reflection on the water seemed to light up the whole place. Maggie listened to the songs of frogs and crickets as a warm mountain breeze started up.

Suddenly, she felt that she was not alone. She looked to the left and right, but she didn't see anyone, even though she felt a presence. Thinking it was her imagination, she tried to let it go, but the more she tried to let it go, the stronger the feeling became.

Maggie stood up and headed back to the ranch. On the way, she noticed a small footbridge over the river. She stood in the middle of the bridge, watching the water and listening to the night sounds. She leaned over the edge rail, watching the white foam forming in the fast water. Then she heard and felt footsteps.

Maggie kept concentrating on the water, but as the footsteps got closer, a feeling welled up in her heart. Her heart raced and seemed to cry, it was so full of joy and longing. Love screamed from her insides. Maggie was so overwhelmed with these mixed feelings that she didn't dare turn around to see who had set them off. As the footsteps passed by, her tears flowed like another small creek, falling into her mouth. She tasted tears of sweet joy.

The footsteps arrived at the end of the bridge and stopped. Then Maggie turned her head just enough to see the shape of an Indian man. She couldn't see him clearly, but felt two hearts recognize each other despite the dark. Neither of them moved or spoke. Finally the man turned and disappeared into the darkness.

Maggie fell to her knees, weak with loneliness and despair. Not really knowing what had just happened, she sat on the bridge feeling as if she'd lost the only person she had ever loved. Her heart ached and her tears kept flowing. A gentle wind caressed her hair and even the frogs and the crickets stopped singing to honor her sorrow. She stood up and looked at the moon. She brought up her hand drum and began a slow beat. An old song came to her lips.

Wha-ta na-sequk

Wha-ta na-sequk

She-wa tog-na-ku

Wha-ta na-sequk

Oh, my grandmother

quiet the pain within

quiet the pain within.

Slowly Maggie walked toward the cabins. Suddenly she broke out in a run, desperate to find Grandfather. When she got to his cabin, he was asleep, but she burst into the room sobbing and fell into his arms. He just held her and cried with her, not even knowing what it was all about. When Maggie was calmer, he got up and made some tea. He had never seen her like this. She looked old, sitting with her head down. As they sipped the tea, she told him what had happened on the bridge. For the first time, he had no advice, no answer. "The only thing I can do for you is a ceremony. Let me get my medicine bundle, and we will pray together." So they prayed. When they were done, Maggie felt better but didn't want to be alone. She slept that night on the floor of her grandfather's room.

In the morning, they were awakened by the breakfast bell. Then the morning meeting began with a ceremony. The Elders sat in a circle and each one spoke as an Eagle feather was passed from one to another. They shared the wisdom of their years. Maggie had to make a conscious effort to pay attention. At the lunch break, she went down to the river to be alone.

In the afternoon the Elders broke into various groups to discuss different subjects. Maggie again tried to pay attention, but try as she could, it was no use. The afternoon seemed to go on forever. When it was over, she went back to her room and fell asleep.

After supper, the people were drumming and singing and having a good time. The weather was perfect. The sun was still shining, the temperature was pleasant and a warm gentle breeze was blowing from the west. The drumming continued well into the night. Even though there were many people around, Maggie had never felt so alone. She wondered, "How can I feel so alone with all these good people here?" But that is exactly what she felt, alone. At home, when she felt lonely, she went to the water because it soothed her pain.

The night was young, so Maggie took her drum again and went to the river. It was dusk, but still light enough to see. As she sat on a rock by the falls, she felt very close to the Creator. She began to sing an honor song to the Creator. She began softly, but soon her voice was strong enough to be heard above the roar of the waterfall.

As she was about to finish the song, she felt a presence again. This time she stood up and turned around. There behind her was the silhouette of the Indian man. They stared at each other for a long time, both trying to recognize the feeling of this pull. Slowly she laid the drum down. The breeze was blowing directly in her hair. He came toward her. Her heart beat faster. The outline of his face looked familiar. He came closer. She felt comfortable. As they approached each other there was a knowing. He held out his hand, she held out hers. As their hands touched, tears of joy streamed down both their faces. Feelings of familiarity flowed between them until they both recognized that they knew each other from somewhere in the past. In this moment, they didn't need any answers. They held each other, letting the silence do all the communicating, letting the feelings that were so long submerged surface again. They both saw another village in another time and gradually remembered their love, the arrival of the Wisdomkeepers, their separation. They stood embracing, letting the Unseen world rebuild the memories, establish the linkages and restore their bond. As they held each other, two Eagles called their names.

Finally he spoke. "Your name was Two Moons and my name was Two Eagles. Do you remember?" She squeezed his hand and nodded. Her eyes were closed. "My name now is Jim Grizzly. I was born on the Blackfoot reservation. My parents died in a car accident. About four months ago, strange things started to happen to me. I accidentally met these Elders and my life hasn't been the same since." When Maggie squeezed his hand as the tears started to trickle down her face, he knew she understood. "I live on a reservation in the north. My family is in a mess. Alcohol has really caused a lot of damage to my people."

All night long they talked. He told her about his reservation and how he grew up. She did the same. She told him her life's story. By the time they got done, they could see the sun on the horizon, shining its golden rays on the mountainside.

As Maggie and Jim ate breakfast, they could only stare at each other. Smiling, eating, and smiling yet again. Grandfather finally showed up and came to sit beside Maggie. When he turned to look at her, his mouth dropped open. Maggie started to cry. Slowly she began to tell him what had happened.

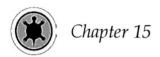 *Chapter 15*

The Prophecies

The drums signaled that the Elders were gathering. Everyone was smudged with sage and one of the Elders offered a prayer. Then another Elder stood and began to speak about the prophecies.

"Last week there was a solar eclipse. This is very significant to Indian people. It fulfills a prophecy from a long time ago. We were told that our people were destined for a cold winter, a time of great difficulty, a time of confusion and hardship. The Old Ones said it would last a long time but it would be over when the sun was blocked in the seventh moon.

"That happened last week, so now the Indian people are entering springtime, a time of healing, a time of brotherhood. This is the coming-together time. During the next twelve moons, the Great Spirit will select the healers. They will be of all colors, all races, all ages. During the coming year, the healers will go through a purification. Many of them will re-examine their lives. They will be searching for the answers to three questions: Who am I? Why am I? Where am I going? They will feel restlessness in their hearts. They will feel that they are supposed to do something, but they won't know what it is.

"When the healing starts, it will happen very quickly. The prophecy says a healing wind will start in the northeast part of Turtle Island. This wind will circle, and when it gains strength, it will blow to the south. Then it will turn and blow west. Then it will turn north once again. This healing wind will touch all the Indian nations."

Maggie gasped, realizing her tribe in the northeast had been given the scrolls for healing.

"During this time a white buffalo calf will be born in the north. This buffalo calf will have the power to bring the people together. Later a Hoop of Eagle feathers will be built. It will have 100 feathers. At this time, Elders from the four directions will be brought together. Elders from the red direction, Elders from the yellow direction, from the black direction and from the white direction. Four ceremonies will be held. In the first ceremony, the people from the red direction will do a ceremony around the Hoop of 100 Eagle Feathers. The Elders will put into the Hoop the power to forgive the unforgivable. Then the Hoop will send that power to all the people of the Earth.

"Next the Elders from the yellow direction will enter the circle and another ceremony will take place, another gift will be sent to the world, the gift of unity. From the black direction the power of healing will come. And finally, from the white direction, the gift of hope. This will be the first time the Elders from all the directions will meet. Their gifts and prayers will bring the people together. It is time for us to become one Earth tribe." Then many other Elders spoke about the prophecies from their tribes. All morning the Elders taught.

During lunch, Jim and Maggie could not eat. They sat by the river as they began to see what their roles would be. They saw very clearly that their purpose was to help heal the Indian communities. Jim and Maggie talked about what they should do. Then they talked to Grandfather and decided Jim would return to the northeast with Grandfather and Maggie.

The Elders continued to teach for four full days. They taught about communities, relationships, and gave many other teachings from the old days.

Home Again, Now What?

The morning after they returned, Maggie stepped outside to offer tobacco, and saw that her brother, the Eagle, was fishing over the water. She liked to watch the male and female Eagles fishing together. She was amazed to watch the male Eagle catch a fish and then fly high with the fish in its claws. When the female Eagle flew underneath him, the male dropped the fish, and his mate caught it in mid air and took it to the young eaglet in their nest. The Eagles had the gift of coordination, of working in balance.

Maggie thought, "This is how Jim and I will work together. We will be like the Eagles and will be mates forever. We will be just like we were in the old village we were taken from." Maggie went inside to shower. She stood under the warm water and realized how happy she was now that Two Eagles was back in her life. She thought about her Grandfather and how grateful she was for his guidance. She wondered what she could say to the community about Jim. She wondered when she would see the Elders again. She wondered if people would listen to her because she was so young. Finally she concluded, "The Creator is in charge, I only need to follow what he says."

As she was cooking, her heart began to pound at the thought of the first breakfast with Jim. She opened a window to let the morning breeze mix with the smell of eggs, fry bread, and coffee. Grandfather and Jim arrived at the door. When her eyes met Jim's, Grandfather's presence faded and only the two of them were there. Jim spoke of how beautiful the village was and how pleased he was to be there. After breakfast, as they sat outside drinking coffee, they heard the Eagle screech high in the sky, and instantly knew they were being called to the cave of the Elders.

As they paddled towards the island, Grandfather told them how little the environment had changed since he was a boy. Only the people had changed. Maggie and Jim just stared at each other. They had so much to talk about, but thus far they had had very little time together. They reached the island and walked in silence to the cave.

They noticed the smell of food cooking on the campfire and the feeling of magic that always seemed to arise in the cave. The Elders welcomed them and soon they were eating their second breakfast. The Elders made small talk, but everyone knew that Maggie and Jim were there for a specific reason.

After the meal, the Elders placed a ceremonial blanket on the ground. They took sage from a medicine bundle and placed it in a shell. Suddenly, Maggie and Jim heard footsteps behind them. They turned to see an old woman wrapped in a white buffalo robe. She had an aura that seemed to glow. Everyone stood up in silence. The new Elder looked warmly at each of them as she approached the campfire. Reaching inside her robe, she brought out two white Eagle fans and laid them on the blanket.

She turned toward Maggie and Jim and motioned for them to come forward. "My name is White Buffalo Calf Woman. Long ago I visited a tribe in the north to bring them a Sacred Pipe. I promised I would return and at that time a great healing would occur and the mending of the hoop would begin. I am keeping my promise. This great healing will occur in the same direction as the destruction, from the east to the west.

"Long ago, both of you were taken from your people because they had and kept the original teachings. When the white man came, we knew he would leave a path of destruction. We knew the time would come when we would have to intervene. We brought you both back at this time to help return the original teachings to the people of the Earth, for the Earth is in very bad shape.

"I am here today to give you a blessing. I am here to join you together, just as you were in the old days. I will perform a traditional marriage ceremony with the Sacred Pipe. When you are married by the pipe, it is forever. Today you will prepare for the ceremony. The men will take you, Jim, and the women will take you, Maggie, to the sacred sweat lodges. In this way you will purify yourselves for the wedding ceremony."

Maggie and Jim looked at each other with tears in their eyes, for they recognized the great honor they were to receive. They followed the Elders to the sweat lodges.

In the evening, Maggie and Jim returned to the cave. A large fire burned, bouncing light off the walls. The smell of sweetgrass filled the cave. Near the fire were two rows of cedar boughs. At the end nearest the fire was a deerskin robe. Maggie was dressed in a traditional white buckskin dress. In the light of the fire, she seemed to glow. The men had given Jim a traditional buckskin outfit that had been passed down from one of the old chiefs. As Jim and Maggie looked at each other, the Eagle's cry echoed throughout the cave.

White Buffalo Calf Woman stood by the fire. Slowly, Maggie and Jim made their way between the rows of cedar branches and knelt on the deerskin. The Elders laid a circle of cedar around them. A drumbeat sounded and the Elders began to sing a very old song. Maggie and Jim held hands. As the song came to a close, White Buffalo Calf Woman reached into her robe and brought out white Eagle feathers and a medicine bag. From the bag, she took a pinch of powder and threw it into the fire. The fire sent up smoke and very colorful flickers. A very warm feeling of love filled the cave. White Buffalo Calf Woman raised the white Eagle feathers and began chanting the marriage blessing. As the feathers were held above their heads, the people were astonished to see golden rays emerge from the white light around the couple, and spread to cover everyone there.

After the blessing, White Buffalo Calf Woman took Maggie and Jim by their right hands, stood them up and said, "Today, you will start a journey which will help heal the world. You have been given special powers. In order for these powers to work, you must work and think like the mated Eagles. This night you are joined as one. You are man and wife."

White Buffalo Calf Woman turned them around to face the other Elders. While they stood there, Grandfather and the Elders slowly left the cave. It was finally time for the newlyweds to be alone.

Early the next morning, Maggie and Jim came out of the cave to offer tobacco. They said a prayer to the Creator and thanked him for bringing them back together. They prayed for the people and for each of them to be obedient to his will. They returned to the cave and Maggie cooked their breakfast.

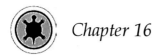 *Chapter 16*

The More Humble You Are, the Greater Leader You Are

Jim and Maggie were canoeing with no particular destination in mind. As they came around a point on Deer Island, they saw a canoe that seemed to be adrift. Going closer, they saw a body slumped over. When they reached it, Maggie recognized Toby, one of the tribal council members. He had passed out once again from too much drink. Jim and Maggie towed the canoe to shore, built a fire and laid Toby on a blanket to make him as comfortable as possible. Meanwhile, Maggie told Jim about Toby.

"A long time ago, Toby was one of our most traditional people. He was raised the traditional way. He was one of our council members and everyone respected him. When the government came to recruit men to go to Vietnam, Toby signed up. He believed it was the calling of the warrior to protect his people. The community gave him an Eagle feather the day he left. He was gone about two years. Something must have happened to him in the war, because they say he was different when he came back. He was restored to the tribal council, but he quit participating in the traditions. He wouldn't attend ceremonies, not even any social events. And he started to drink. Everyone in the community still loved him, but he became a prisoner of that bottle.

"Toby was born into one of the reservation's bigger clans," Maggie continued. "The bigger the clan, the more likely the clan can vote in who they want when it comes to tribal election. Even though Toby drank too much, he always ran for tribal elections and he always won. The problem is when Toby was drinking, he would agree to anything anybody said. He wouldn't create any conflict. He would vote according to what he told the last person. He has a wife, Nina, and two children, but sometimes he disappears for days or even weeks. Nina is just waiting for him to quit drinking, she says she'll never give up on him, but he won't even talk to her about what's going on with him. He was always very quiet. I think he wants to quit but he can't. He's become a prisoner of the bottle and doesn't think much of himself."

Jim listened until Maggie had told the whole story. Then he spoke. "I know what you mean. My reservation is the same. Alcohol is destroying the lives of all our people. The people are destroying themselves." Toby stirred and the smell of alcohol filled the air. His face was bloated and his clothes dirty; he probably hadn't eaten for several days. Maggie brought food from the canoe and began to prepare a meal.

When the smell of coffee was in the air, Toby sat up feeling sick and hungover. His head ached from too much alcohol. Maggie introduced Jim. Toby said he was glad to meet him, but he was in too much pain to make much conversation. Maggie handed him a plate of food and he slowly began to eat. After they finished the silent meal, Maggie went down to the lake and came back with a wet cloth to help Toby clean up. As she began to wash his face, Toby broke out in deep sobs. Maggie and Jim sat near him in silence. Finally he was calm enough to speak. "I am so ashamed. I have disgraced my people, my family and myself. I no longer have the ability to lead the people. I am nothing. I can't quit drinking. I am going to die a loser."

Maggie and Jim didn't try to talk with Toby then. They recognized he needed to be alone. They brought a tent and a sleeping bag from their canoe, set up the tent and left all the food they had. As they paddled away, Maggie wept because she knew Toby before the war must have been a proud Indian man, connected with his people, his culture, and the Creator. Jim quietly paddled back to the island of the Elders' cave.

The Elders returned that night as Maggie and Jim lay listening to the fire. Maggie prepared food as usual, but the Elders sensed something was bothering her. Shining Star came to her, pulled up her sad face and asked her what was wrong. Tears welled up in Maggie's eyes as she related the story about Toby. When she was done, Shining Star hugged her and told her not to worry. The evening fire died away about the same time they all got into their blankets to sleep.

In the morning Maggie noticed there was another person in a blanket close to the fire. She moved closer and recognized Toby. Looking around for an explanation, she saw Shining Star with a slight smile on her face. When Toby finally woke up, he was startled. The Elders were sitting in council, speaking a language he had never heard. He thought he was dreaming. But when Shining Star looked at him, he knew it was real. Two of the Elders moved aside and invited Toby into the circle. Toby was afraid.

The Elder spoke. "Toby, we are the Elders from the Wisdomkeepers. Don't be afraid. We are here to help your people. A great healing is going to occur among the Indian nations. Your village is chosen as the place where the healing wind will start. As your community heals, it will generate a healing wind. This wind will become very strong. Soon the wind will blow across Turtle Island. It will leave your community and first blow south, then it will blow to the west and finally to the north. This healing wind will bring a Wellbriety Movement to all Indian nations. Your community will be healed and, in return, will help other Indian nations to heal. We have been watching your community and your leaders. We know you have all forgotten the old ways. When you were young, your grandfather taught you, but you went to the war of the white man and your spirit is wounded. We are here to help you heal your spirit so you can quit drinking and begin to help your people. We will do a ceremony for you. We will give you a medicine pouch to keep around your neck. You will not remember what is going on now, but you will be healed and empowered to lead your people."

In the background a drum started to beat and Toby heard the Elders singing. He closed his eyes as the song made his heart remember the teachings of the old people. The Elders began the ceremony to rid Toby of the evil spirit he had picked up during the war. He screamed as the spirit struggled out of his body. Then Toby fell over onto his side and into a deep sleep.

In the morning, Toby woke up outside the tent, back on Deer Island. As the sun shone on his face, he sensed something was different. He crawled to the water to look at his reflection. His eyes were different, no longer cold. He didn't feel numb anymore. He sat down on a rock and noticed a weight around his neck. He grasped the medicine bag and sat there quite a while, wondering how he might have received it. He knew he sometimes blacked out when he drank and that his memory was unreliable. He kept the bag around his neck.

Toby struck the tent, packed it into his canoe, and headed back to the village. As he paddled, he felt a newness, a freshness he had not felt in many years. The hole he had carried inside was gone. For the first time in years, he sang a traditional paddling song. Suddenly a shadow covered him. He looked up just as an Eagle flew over his head, so close he could have touched it. Tears of joy flowed down his cheeks as he paddled faster. He didn't know, or even need to know, what had happened to him, except that he had been healed.

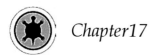 *Chapter17*

Toby's Vision

Toby got home early that morning, but his wife and children had already left for work and school. He was glad to be alone in his new state of mind. He showered, scraped together some breakfast, and then set out for the tribal office and the daily council meeting. In the past, if he went at all, he would trudge along, eyes on the ground. But now he looked up and noticed the beauty of the land he had formerly taken for granted. Toby closed his eyes and inhaled as he walked along the path. The air was pure and fresh. For the first time he heard many birds singing. When he saw the usual group of Elders visiting by the community wood pile, he greeted them with such warmth that they were startled. As he passed by, the older ones who remembered his younger years remarked that he seemed to be more like the man they knew before the war.

As Toby approached the tribal offices, he heard bits of gossip from people along the way. Jake Old Crow, the tribe's lieutenant governor was in jail. This wasn't unusual: on most weekends, two or more of the council got in trouble for something or other. Everyone on the council drank, so it was no surprise that Jake had got drunk and beaten his wife. Outside the council chamber, Toby heard the council members arguing. When he entered the room, everyone fell silent. They were a bit surprised to see him, but they were stunned by how he had changed. Toby simply filled his coffee cup and sat down in his usual chair. No one said a word to him. As they resumed the discussion, Toby looked around at his fellow council members.

The five members and the tribal Governor, Gib Doxtator, were there. Only Jake Old Crow was missing. Toby listened as the meeting picked up momentum. Soon the usual arguing and bickering escalated into a shouting match about whose relative should get a new job at the health department. Each council member was promoting his own relative or pushing his personal agenda. Toby listened with a different pair of ears this morning. He decided to sit and listen and not to enter any discussion unless he was asked. By noon he hadn't said a word.

The council meeting ended without decisions. Toby left the building and slowly walked through the village, feeling sad. Previously, he would have spent the rest of the day without thinking much about the meeting, but now he wondered why the leaders acted as they did. He continued walking, noticing the people, the tone of their voices, and how their body language revealed their feelings. He heard children crying and adults shouting hateful things at them. He smelled marijuana and saw that the children had no glow in their eyes. The teenagers glanced indifferently at him and the younger children held their heads low. He saw houses with yards full of junk cars and windows broken out, sometimes taped but seldom repaired. He saw doors that had been kicked in anger. He saw the bruised face of a once-beautiful woman who had stayed too long with her abusive husband. He heard curses and disrespect among the teenagers. He felt the despair and hopelessness of the people. He remembered having the same feelings of desperation in Vietnam and began to cry.

Toby went to a place by the river, close to where it met the ocean. Long ago it had been his secret spot where he could sit and let his thoughts flow downstream. He knew when you were troubled if you sat by the water, the water spirits would take your troubles away. The water soothed his feelings and cleared his mind as he imagined his troubles flowing to the sea. It was a clear day and Shellback Island was visible in the distance. Toby thought it would be good to spend the night there. His uncle had taken him to the island a number of times when he was a young child. The island was a place of calm and magic. He remembered how vivid his imagination could be. He used to call it his dream place. He went home and packed some food and warm clothes. As he was loading them into his canoe, one of the village Elders, Sam Yellow Eagle, stopped by. Sam saw that Toby had changed, but said nothing about his observation. He simply asked where Toby might be going. When Toby mentioned Shellback Island, Sam told him that long ago it had been the place for warriors to fast and seek visions. Toby had great respect for Sam. He watched the old man gesture with his wrinkled hand. Sam told him the cliff on the east side of the island had a sacred altar the people had used to seek their visions. It was as if Sam was giving him special, secret instructions. Toby thanked him and set off.

He thought about his people as he paddled. What could he do to help them? As the island came into view, he decided to find the sacred altar and camp on the cliff. He came ashore and set out up the steep hill, the smell of salt water still in the air. At length, he reached the top of the cliff. It didn't take much effort to see the sacred place. The altar stones were still there, but they were overgrown with grasses and had clearly not been used for many years. Toby set up his simple camp, then sat down on a rock and gazed at the altar. He imagined his ancestors using it. An hour later, he was still focused on the altar, but he had begun to feel restless. The feeling came from inside, as if he was supposed to do something. Ordinarily, Toby would have discounted such an intuition, but now he quietly let it build until he recognized the need to pray. It had been such a long time since he prayed, he wasn't sure he could remember what to do.

He gathered some dry branches and fresh cedar and brought them to the altar. He replaced some of the rocks that had fallen from the circle. As he turned away to bring the wood, he noticed tiny spots of color among the rocks beside the fire circle. A beaded medicine pouch lay there, still filled with small bunches of sweetgrass and sage. Toby gently laid the pouch on the altar. He stared at the medicine bag, sensing its power. He had a strong urge to pick it up. In his hand, it felt like part of his body. Toby put it around his neck. Then he strolled to the highest point of the cliff and looked out over the ocean. Even though he was alone on the island, he felt the presence of spirits.

Toby returned to the altar and took off his shirt. He lit a fire. At first the smoke swirled in a dark cloud, but then it rose skyward. Toby knelt and noticed the weight of the medicine bags on his chest. This was the first time he started to think consciously about where the first one had really come from. He took the first, plain, medicine bag from around his neck and held it in his hand. He rolled some of the sage from the beaded medicine pouch into a small ball and lit it in the fire. He put both of his hands around the medicine bags and held them up in the air. As the sage began to burn, the smoke from the wood fire started to swirl like a little tornado. It moved faster and created a big circle. As the smoke circle grew, Toby felt caught up in its motion. He held the medicine bags more tightly as he began to feel that he was falling. It seemed that he was falling through a tunnel in space toward a white light. As he approached the light, he felt safe and loved. When the sensation of movement stopped, he opened his eyes and found himself standing in a beautiful garden.

The garden was filled with birds singing, pleasant smells, and multi-colored flowers. There was a path and he set out on it. It seemed to lead toward the center of the garden. As he approached a clearing, he saw two old people sitting on a log. They seemed to be waiting for him and greeted him with smiles. The old woman asked Toby what they could do to help him. Toby was puzzled. He sensed that these two Elders were really special and he wanted to share his innermost feelings about his people. Toby told them, "My people are dying. We are in trouble. I am a tribal leader but I don't know how I can help." He felt no need to explain in detail—he sensed the Elders knew much more than he did.

The Elders looked at each other in silence. Slowly, the old woman got up and left. In a few minutes, she returned with a strange pouch made of deerskin and handed it to the old man. He untied the pouch and pulled out a long roll of birch bark. He unrolled it and placed it in front of Toby. On the scroll were ten symbols. Toby looked at them carefully, then he slowly looked up at the Elders. The old man spoke.

"Within these symbols are the secret knowledge of leadership. Take this scroll with you. Use your medicine bags to pray. Do this and you will help your people. Go in peace."

Toby rolled up the scroll and put it back into the deerskin pouch. He bowed respectfully to the Elders as he left the clearing. On the way back he saw a little pond. There he sat on a rock to think about what had just happened. He leaned forward to see his reflection. As he gazed at it, he could see that he was a different person. Suddenly, the pond became the opening of a cave and Toby tumbled in. He fell for a long time.

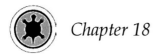 *Chapter 18*

Reading the Scrolls

Toby realized he was lying on the ground. He heard crickets chirping and the distant call of a whip-poor-will, so he knew it was night. He opened his eyes and saw by the moonlight that he was back at the cliff on Shellback Island. He got up and built a fire. The flames lit the altar and a large deerskin pouch lying there. This pouch was tanned, with long fringes and a shoulder strap. He picked it up and took out the scroll of ten symbols. Toby clutched the scroll to his chest as he remembered where it came from. He knelt and offered thanks that his prayer for a way to help the people had been answered. He felt close to nature and to the Creator. His heart was warm.

In the morning, Toby packed his canoe and headed back to the village. As he approached the shore, he saw that an ordinary day was in full swing. Children were playing in the schoolyard. The morning was filled with birds singing, the dogs were playing their games, some of the people were standing around catching up on the latest gossip, and others were walking with a pace that showed they had purpose to their journey. The air was fresh with the morning odors of breakfast and flowers.

When The Student Is Ready

Jim and Maggie were building a traditional sweat lodge with a group of young people. They had gathered willow poles and were placing them in the ground to form a framework for the lodge. Toby came by and mentioned he was glad to see them taking an interest in this traditional practice. Maggie said that if Toby wanted to sweat with them, she, Jim and Toby would have the first sweat in the new lodge. Toby said he would be honored to pray with them and joined them in finishing the lodge. They built it carefully with the door in the east. The sixteen willow poles were placed precisely and bent to make the body of the lodge perfect. Carefully they bound the willows with red cloth. Then they covered the lodge with blankets and arranged the altar outside the lodge and the fire pit inside. They understood that the sweat lodge symbolized the womb of mother earth, the altar represented the moon, and the fire pit symbolized the sun. The entire story of the universe and how man fits into it is demonstrated in the design of the sweat lodge. This knowledge existed with the Elders since the beginning of time.

That evening, the young people built a fire to heat the rocks. Traditionally, when Native youths first become interested in using the sweat lodge, their first duties will be to build the fire to heat the rocks. When Toby arrived, Maggie and Jim were ready. The three of them got into the lodge, and the fire tender brought the heated rocks, one at a time, on a shovel. The first seven were placed in the fire pit at the center of the lodge while everyone remained silent. The rocks are called Grandfathers. They are so old that they know all things. Jim sprinkled each one with cedar and the lodge filled with fragrant smoke. Then the door flap was closed and the lodge became completely dark. Toby heard the sound of water hitting the rocks and a wave of hot steam struck him as the prayer songs began. They prayed in a pitiful way, asking for help for all the people. After several songs, the door flap was opened and more rocks were brought in for the second round. When Toby began to pray, Maggie was startled to hear him asking for understanding of the symbols he had received on his prayer journey to the island. Maggie's heart beat faster and Jim could sense her excitement. She could hardly keep her focus during the rest of the sweat. Maggie understood how Toby might have received the scrolls, but she would have a thousand questions to ask him after the sweat.

When they finished, Maggie asked Toby to come to her home, but she kept silent as the three of them walked together. When they arrived at her house, Maggie made coffee, then sat down and asked Toby about the symbols he had prayed about. Toby brought out the deerskin pouch and showed the scroll to Maggie. Maggie was delighted to see the symbols. She went into her bedroom and came back with the ten pouches the Elders had given her. She told Toby how she had received them. She gave Toby the first scroll and the same instructions the Elders gave her about reading the scroll four times each day. Toby was to come to her when he was ready for the second one.

Reading Scroll One

~ *Change Is From Within* ~

Toby considered the instructions as he read through the first scroll. "This is strange," he thought. No one had ever told him that repetition is one of the ways to learn. But he decided to give it a try. Early next morning, Toby awoke as usual, but he read the scroll aloud as part of his morning meditation and resolved to do the reading four times each day.

At nine O'clock, Toby arrived at the tribal offices. Jake Old Crow sat in his usual place, but barely nodded as Toby walked by. Toby made coffee as the other council members arrived. When the council was assembled, Gib Doxtator wrote the morning's agenda on a blackboard. Two council members who had drunk up their paychecks asked to be on the agenda so they could get money to feed their children. Another member was trying to get an allotment of land for her cousin who was moving back to the reservation. Four members of the tribe wanted to attend a conference on child abuse in Washington State, but there was only enough money for two. The meeting got started, along with the usual bickering. When they started in on the land allotment, the arguing got worse and more personal. Each member fought for his own opinion. Toby tried to step in, but the entire council and a few of the tribal members turned on him. "Who the hell do you think you are, you drunk? We've put up with you and your drunkenness for years while you just sat like a bump on a log. Now you want to get into the act? You think you can play the peacemaker and take care of our business, but you don't even take care of your own." Toby was offended and struck back by reminding the council members of their own failings. The verbal brawl continued with occasional interruptions from tribe members wanting to get their electricity turned on, or needing gas money, or lodging various complaints. Members of the tribe were allowed to attend all meetings except executive sessions, so the people took the opportunity to express their anger and frustration. The meetings were stressful and the bickering and backbiting were ferocious.

At the lunch break, Toby headed for his spot near the water. He sat there a while, feeling frustrated and angry, but when he looked up and saw the island, he remembered his commitment to read the scroll. He took it out and studied the image of a buffalo with an arrow pointing within. "I must be the change I wish to see . . . Real power is in knowing myself . . . Oh Great Spirit, teach me to change myself . . ." As Toby read the scroll with the painful memory of the council meeting fresh in his mind, he realized how he had been contributing to the problem. He used to roll his eyes and shake his head sarcastically. He would sit in the council meeting without really participating, but judging and gossiping in his mind.

Toby realized he hadn't even remembered the scroll during the morning. Toby thought about the scroll. "It says I need to change myself first, I need to establish contact with the Great Spirit and let him guide me through the conflict." He sat quietly for the rest of the hour, then slowly walked back to the tribal offices.

During the afternoon session, Toby began to notice how he was giving his power away. If someone criticized him, his first impulse was to attack them in return. If they gossiped about him, he gossiped back. If he wanted to get even with someone, he would spread a rumor. All afternoon there was tension and fighting. Finally the council called an executive session, and the people left.

That evening after the kids were settled in bed and his wife was doing her nightly chores, Toby read the scroll again, and he read it once more before he went to sleep. "I must be the change..."

During the next several weeks, Toby continued to read the scroll four times each day and his insight about how he let other people determine his behavior continued to grow. Sometimes he would carry resentment all day long, or he would think about revenge. He realized that he was backstabbing and gossiping when he actually needed to handle the conflict in a straightforward manner. As he continued to work with the scroll, he began to see that he could change his response if, each time he was irritated, he remembered to talk to the Creator. He began to see that if he wanted to receive respect, he needed to offer respect to others. He could continue to take things personally, or he could understand that people were acting out of fear and hurt.

Now when the council was arguing and fighting, Toby would center himself. After some practice, he could consistently settle his mind in this way. By the fourth week, the council members noticed they couldn't hit his buttons. They began asking for his opinion. They could see his words had spiritual meanings. He was becoming a peacemaker in the council and other groups in the community were asking him to stop in and help. Finally Toby came to understand the power of the first scroll.

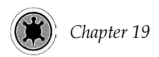 *Chapter 19*

You Must Be the Change You Wish to See

In every community there are people who criticize anyone who tries to make a positive change. It is like the "crab bucket syndrome." If one of the crabs starts to climb out of the bucket, the others will try to pull it back in. As Toby began to change himself, as he tried to be positive and get his life back together, Jake Old Crow got jealous. Toby used to drink and raise the roof with him. They had been drinking partners on the reservation and in the neighboring towns. Now Jake started to spread rumors about Toby. He told stories to undermine Toby's credibility in the community, and he even told stories that could harm Toby's family. He said Toby's wife was running around with other men. He said Toby had women friends in the cities and that he was sleeping around. He spread rumors that Toby had used tribal funds to finance his drinking sprees.

Some of the community members believed these stories. Eventually they circulated a petition to remove him from the council. If they gathered 250 signatures, the council would have to hold an investigative session to find out if the allegations were true. And if they were, then a special election would have to be held. Because Toby had only recently stopped drinking, people didn't know what to believe. When they saw him walking through the village, some turned away and others jeered at him.

One evening as Toby was walking by the water, he encountered Jake, who had been drinking. When Jake saw him, he staggered toward Toby, gesturing wildly and shouting. Toby had had enough. He grabbed the Lt. Governor by the collar.

"Enough of this positive-thinking crap," he thought. Just as he raised his fist to punch Jake, the birch bark scroll fell out of his pocket and he was faced with a choice between the old way and the new one. He let Jake go, picked up the scroll, and continued his walk.

When the investigative meeting was held, Jake got up and repeated his accusations. Then, one by one, members of the community stood up and expressed their confidence in Toby. The council determined the allegations were false, and Toby retained his seat. Toby realized the importance of prayer and of becoming the change he wished to see in the community.

Reading Scroll Two

~ Use The Powers Of The East ~

The second full moon had arrived so it was time to get the next scroll. Toby talked with Jim and Maggie about how many times he wanted to give up and how the scroll didn't seem to have anything to do with what was going on. But he had seen how reading the scroll repeatedly started an internal conflict. Then, through the conflict, his understanding of the scroll developed. He understood this was necessary for his beliefs to change. Now he could simply look at the symbol and automatically shift his mind to the place of guidance. He knew that when he became irritated it was best to find that place before speaking.

Maggie received the first scroll and offered Toby the second one. He quietly accepted the pouch. Now that he knew their effects, he had more respect for the scrolls.

When he got home, the children were asleep and his wife, Nina, was getting ready for bed. She lightly touched his arm as he entered the kitchen. She had been so proud of him this past month. She had prayed for him so many years and finally her prayers were being answered. Toby looked at his wife. Her Grandmother called her Still Water, because she was always so calm. Toby always knew he would marry her. Even when she was a little girl, he knew from the way she looked at him that she would want to be his wife.

He could see the love she had for him in her eyes. He loved her eyes when she looked at him in this special way. He touched her cheek and she closed her eyes, for she had always known he loved her, too. When she saw he had another scroll, she knew he needed to be alone. Toby lit some sage to purify himself and unrolled the scroll. At the top of the scroll was a symbol that looked like the rising sun. Toby looked at it for a long time before he started to read. "Use the powers of the east . . ."

When he had finished, he carefully replaced the scroll in its pouch, then walked to the door and looked at the full moon. For the first time he felt human, knew he was fully alive. He went outside and sat down. When he touched the medicine bag around his neck, chills ran through his fingers. "Why have I been chosen for this?" he wondered. Feeling a need to pray, he got some tobacco from the house offered it in thanks for his life to the Great Mystery.

Toby woke at dawn, built a fire and prepared sage and tobacco for the morning ceremony. Silently, he waited for sunrise, trying to keep his mind quiet as it raced in anticipation of the morning sun.

Be still . . . Be still . . . Be still . . . Soon the horizon colored up with different shades of pink and rose. Toby held his medicine bag in his hand and stood facing east as the sun appeared over the horizon. When the first sunbeams struck his face, the medicine pouch began to vibrate. He closed his eyes as his senses responded to the gifts of the east. He heard birds singing and found he could distinguish one bird's song from another. He heard breezes moving through the trees and began to feel connected to them. He opened his eyes and watched the shape of the sun form a complete circle as it rose above the horizon. He read the scroll aloud and called upon the powers of the east. On his way back to the house, he felt like a new person walking hand in hand with the universe.

Toby ate a hearty breakfast and set out for work. His mind was full of the morning's experience. He felt close to the Creator. He felt connected, but his thoughts were interrupted by the flashing lights of the tribal police car parked near the office building. Toby walked faster toward the small groups of people who were standing around as usual, but they looked distressed and were talking quietly among themselves. One of the Little Bear family's teenaged sons had committed suicide. Toby knew the family very well and this news shocked him badly. He went directly to his office to call the family, who lived some distance from the village, but their phone was busy or off the hook. He sat at his desk, feeling deeply saddened, not only because of this tragedy but because there had been two other teen suicides in the past several months. The community had been upset, but nothing had yet been done to address the problem.

When the council had all arrived, the governor called a short meeting to address the community concerns. As usual, the council was at a loss about how to handle the aftermath of suicides. They called a day of mourning out of respect for the family and because they knew all the tribal employees would call in sick. Soon the telephone started to ring with calls from people wanting to know what the council was going to do about the problem. After a few of these calls, they let the answering machine take over and sat drinking coffee and talking the usual small talk until they were startled by the sound of a gunshot. It seemed to have come from the tribal housing behind the council building. When they got to the back door, a woman's screams were coming from the middle house. Some of the neighbors were already at the open door. Anna stood inside, covered with blood. As one of the neighbor women embraced her, she fell to her knees, sobbing. A man gently stepped past her into the next room and immediately came out vomiting. Anna's son was Joe Little Bear's best friend, and he, too, had just shot himself.

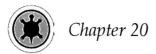 *Chapter 20*

The Power of the Circle

The council just stood there, dumbfounded, until someone mentioned the local tavern. Toby tried to get them back to the council room, but they knew they couldn't handle the pressure of people coming to them for help in yet another emergency when they themselves didn't know what to do. They were going to get drunk.

Even though Toby had seen many deaths in the community, he was devastated. A normal death was bad enough, but when a teenager committed suicide, it paralyzed the community. When the community froze, the teenagers isolated themselves in clusters. And in those tight groups, suicide pacts were sometimes made. Toby was afraid of losing more teenagers. He walked to his place by the water and sat on a rock, letting his thoughts go downstream. The glare of the sun on the water reminded him it was noon and time for the second scroll. "Use the powers of the east . . . " After the reading, Toby reflected on how centered he had been in the morning and how disturbed he was now, only a few hours later. He faced the east, took the medicine bag from his neck, held it in his outstretched hand, and sang a traditional healing song for his people. Tears rolled down his face and his heart was full of hurt and loneliness as his voice echoed the water. HIA-WU-NA-NUK-QUICHS-SAH.

Toby was desperate. The community was in crisis, the council was off drinking, and he didn't know what to do. As he held the medicine bag to his heart. he realized that the people were afraid and they should gather in a circle to support each other and talk about their feelings. As this thought ran through his mind, he heard an eagle screech and knew what he was to do.

Toby went back to the largest room at the tribal center and arranged the chairs in a circle. He went to the courtyard behind the building and asked a few of the youth gathered there to go around the community and inform the people that a talking circle would be taking place. Within a half hour, a hundred people had arrived. Toby laid a red cloth in the center of the circle and lit a bowl of sage. After everyone had been smudged, he took an Eagle feather, placed it over his heart and began to speak. He talked about his fears, his anger, his doubt about the Creator, and his love for everyone in the community. When there was nothing left in his heart to say, when every emotion had been expressed out loud to the circle, when he had fully opened himself to everyone and had no words remaining, he passed the feather to the person on his left. All afternoon the people talked, sobbed, wailed, and wept. Toby listened. Some people were hysterical, some were in despair.

When the feather had gone around two or three times, people began to calm down. Someone asked what could be done to help the bereaved families and the young people who had no hope for the future. Toby was discouraged, especially because the leadership was off drinking. But as he listened to the people, he began to see that the power of the circle was working. When one person took the risk of sharing his innermost self, it became easier for the next person to do the same. Many people shared what they had felt and done when they, too, had lost loved ones. Some expressed how they were able to turn tragedy into help for others. They learned things about one another that they hadn't known before, even though they all lived in the same community and worked together every day. As the people began to trust the power of the circle, the conversation turned to what they could do.

Toby started taking notes as people came up with ideas. He asked for volunteers, two Elders, four adults, and four youths, to join him in a circle of creative thinkers. "We will be the calm ones. We will be the responsible ones. We will be the stability until this is over. We will make a plan to get us through this crisis."

They called the director of mental health and arranged to have counselors available around the clock. Talking circles would be held every four hours, from early morning to late evening. Counseling was to be available at several locations to anyone affected by the suicides, including tribal police who had been called to the scenes, friends and relatives. Special talking circles were set up to explain things to the very young. They established a community crisis line. But not every household had a phone, so they had the youth deliver the critical information. Each of them was responsible for a certain group of houses. In this way, the youth became the communication link. Many of them began to feel like part of the community for the first time. When they delivered information to the houses, the people shook their hands and thanked them for helping. Sometimes they were invited in to eat. The youths were glad to be involved in helping. They distributed suicide prevention information, so people would know what signs to watch for and who to call for help. The people were told to notice if their children were isolating themselves, drinking, acting secretive, talking about leaving their possessions to someone, or saying goodbye to brothers and sisters or friends. Every youth was located. Their families and friends helped identify those who might be at risk. Then the Elders remembered an ancient healing ceremony and offered to conduct it the day after the funerals.

The families held the funerals together because the two boys had been such good friends. The entire community showed up. There was no longer any hysteria, but a cloud of sadness hung over the entire village. At the end of the funeral, the Elders put a red mark on everyone's cheek to signify that you had accepted that the deceased had gone to the spirit world and was now with the Creator. They now belonged to him.

Early the next morning, the people gathered for the healing ceremony. They stood in a line while the drum sounded slowly. The four Elders stood in pairs across from one another. One held sage, one carried water, one held sweetgrass, and the other had an Eagle fan. Four pipe carriers prayed to the four directions. Many people in the community were surprised to see that there were still some people who knew the old ways. As the drumbeat picked up, the people walked between the pipe carriers and then between the Elders who blessed them with water, smudged them with sage and sweetgrass, and finally touched them with the Eagle feather. As the people passed through this tunnel of healing, they joined hands in a circle. When the last person joined the circle, the rhythm of the drum changed and the people began a round dance with the Elders praying and the pipe carriers pointing their pipes to the Creator in the center of the circle. The drum got louder and the people danced harder, held on to each other's hands more tightly, and started to feel the healing. They looked on one another with loving eyes and hearts. They danced back and forth for an hour. When the drum stopped, they hugged one another. Toby danced and watched. This was the first time he had seen the community expressing their love for each other. The crisis was over.

Toby and Nina walked home silently, hand in hand. They were exhausted. Nina went immediately to bed while Toby locked up the house and sat down to read the scroll. He began to understand its lessons.

When you are afraid and don't know what to do, face the east and
grasp the hand of the Great Spirit.

When the people need help, there are powers to assist if you ask
the Grandfathers for help.

There is a voice inside that will guide you.

The Ancestors are within.

Toby crawled into bed, looked at his sleeping wife, kissed her
on the cheek, and collapsed on his pillow.

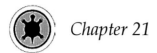 *Chapter 21*

Conflict

Toby continued to read the scroll four times each day. Every day he had new insights and understandings. He knew he could connect with the power in the morning, but it was difficult to stay with it during the day because there was so much conflict. He wasn't always able to stay centered. On the full moon, Maggie brought the scroll about the powers of the south.

Toby spent the first week reading the scroll as usual, but now he watched his reactions and observed how other people were responding. He wondered about the connection between conflict and resolution. Often, if someone upset him, he would be irritated or doubtful. Then he would figure out how to get even, or how to get rid of the irritating person. If he acted on that, then he would have to be on guard, because the person would be planning how to get even with him. He was caught in a cycle of conflict and revenge and he couldn't see how to break it.

Reading Scroll Three

~ *Use The Powers Of The South* ~

Toby went to the island to spend a day alone. He wanted to meditate on the new scroll. It was a clear day and, as he approached the island, he noticed a cove he had never visited. He paddled to shore and as he was tying the canoe to a rock he saw a large, unusual shell. He picked it up and carried it to a group of rocks that stood between the beach and the forest. There he laid out an altar, placing the shell and his medicine bag in the center. He sat on the ground facing the south and smudged himself with sweetgrass. The fragrance was soothing. Toby closed his eyes. He felt the breeze blowing his hair and the warmth of the sun. His mind began to settle down. He focused on the breeze for he knew the wind was the voice of the Great Spirit. The wind whispered a soothing, low hum. Toby became drowsy. He opened his eyes and saw the shell. It seemed to be getting bigger. It grew until its opening looked like the mouth of a cave.

On the wall of the cave, Toby noticed a painting of a patch of flowers. It seemed to be moving. He watched more closely and saw that the plants were growing rapidly. In a few minutes he had seen their entire development from seed to a bare stem, to a stem with leaves. He saw how a bulb develops and watched the bulb send up a shoot and unfold a flower. He saw how flowers produce seeds, which fall back to the earth as the flowers wither and die.

Then Toby heard the wind speak, "Become the seed." Toby imagined being a seed and felt the pain of growth. The insides of the seed turned to muck and the new roots struggled downward through the soil, seeking moisture. At the same time, the new stem fought upward toward the light. It was very painful.

Finally, the stem broke through the soil and there was a period of relief, but the pain returned as the stem began to send out leaves. Then Toby felt some relief until the stem tip became a bud. The development of the bud was very stressful and painful. As Toby felt the conflict of growth, he sensed it was part of a natural process. Soon the stress of change resumed as the bud grew larger. Excitement exploded throughout Toby's being as the bud opened into a flower. He felt the presence of the great life force with all its beauty and love. Then he knew he was to produce seeds so the life cycle would continue. He felt release and sadness. Soon the seeds dropped and he felt himself going on to the other side.

Toby found himself looking at the painting as the wind asked, "What did you learn from this experience?" Toby sat in silence, listening to the voice within.

For Anything To Grow or Change,
it Must First Struggle To Do So First.

Conflict And Struggle Are Part Of The Natural Order.

Conflict Precedes Clarity.

Nature Is The Final Teacher.

Toby turned and left the cave.

Suddenly, he sat up as a light rain shower started. He looked around. It was no longer sunny and he could tell it was near evening, so he headed back to the village. As he paddled across the water, he thought about the community conflicts and tried to see them as signs of growth.

Toby continued to read the scroll, wondering how its teachings could be applied in the community. Each day he attended the morning councils. Each day there were conflicts and arguments. One day as he sat at his spot near the water, an Elder came strolling by. It was Joe Porcupine who conducted many of the tribal ceremonies and had great insight to the Spirit World. People often sought him out to interpret their dreams.

Toby asked what he thought was the reason for the strife in the community. Joe told him, "There are two great enemies in our village. One enemy is alcohol and the other enemy is jealousy. These two enemies keep us fighting. Because we have abandoned our ceremonies and culture, we no longer know how to live in harmony. We no longer build relationships with each other."

And he went on. "There are four ways to handle conflict. First, when conflict occurs, we can attack one another. Second, when conflict occurs, we can withhold from one another. We can keep information to ourselves, we can avoid going to meetings. Third, we can deny there is a problem. For example, we know our community has a lot of sexual abuse going on, but we all pretend it's not a problem. We pretend alcohol is not a big problem. Fourth, we can embrace conflict. We can look at it, we can admit it is real, we can acknowledge the problem and sit down together to find a solution. The solution is inside the conflict."

Toby was amazed at how simple it was once Joe had explained. He asked Joe to speak about the four directions of conflict at the next council. When he did, Toby could see the principles made sense to the other council members, but there were questions about how they could actually be put to use. The Elder had the council sit in a circle. He wrote on four pieces of paper, saying "First you choose which one you want to use."

He held up the first word, "attack," showing it to each council member. "Will you choose to solve conflict in this way? Do you want to attack each other whenever a conflict occurs? Please raise your hands if this is your choice." The circle was silent and no hands were raised.

"How many of you will withhold or run when conflict occurs? Raise your hands." There was no response.

Holding up the third word, "deny," he asked, "How many of you want to pretend we don't have a problem? Raise your hands." Silence again.

"How many of you are willing to learn how to embrace the conflict?" Slowly, the council all raised their hands.

"All right," Joe said. "Here's how you go about it. Whenever two or more of you are gathered, pray. It's more important to pray than to do anything else at the beginning."

"Then let your decisions be for the people first, yourselves last."

"If you get a conflict going, stop and light the sage or sweet grass. Then you should all meditate. Be silent for a few minutes. Take the Eagle feather and let everyone talk. Then vote for what is best for the community."

"Do this for six months. Give it a chance."

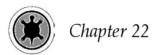 *Chapter 22*

Toby Learns About Letting Go

Toby finished the third scroll. As he thought about it each day, he began to see that conflict actually did precede clarity. He developed new ways of understanding conflict. As soon as a conflict arose, he set his mind on the principle of conflict and refrained from judging people, especially when they were emotional. Even when people attacked him, he could see that every attack was a cry out for love. Over the thirty days with the scroll, he saw that the council members were working better together. And he saw himself developing an eagle's point of view about the community. He was ready to read the next scroll.

Reading Scroll Four

~ Use The Powers Of The West ~

Lakota Elder Frank Fools Crow once said, *The two greatest enemies Native people have are Number 1, alcohol, and Number 2, jealousy.* If we are maintaining resentments and grudges day after day, eventually these resentments block us from making good decisions. It is so important for our leaders to clear these feelings up each day so we are able to maintain the good mind.

Maggie saw Toby sitting by the water's edge one evening so she delivered the next scroll. They talked about the difficulty of living in a community dominated by negativity and jealousy. The tide was coming in, splashing the shells and old sea grass lying on the beach. The beach got dirty during the day and the water cleaned it up at night. After Maggie left, Toby unrolled the fourth scroll and read through it very carefully. The power of the west was about letting go and reviewing one's actions at the end of each day. Toby went home and was still thinking about the scroll as he fell asleep and began to dream.

Toby was standing in a creek with water up to his waist. He lifted his face to the sun, sensed its warmth and brightness through closed eyes, and felt that he was standing in the power of the Creator. His thoughts were clear and his mind was at peace. He heard a splash upstream and was startled to see six small people shoving a big boulder into the water. The little people watched Toby's reaction. Toby was a little excited, but he just stood there and stared back at them. One of the little people grabbed a big tree stump and threw it into the water next to the big rock. Again, the little people stared at Toby. Then they threw another big boulder into the water and stood watching Toby. Toby was getting irritated. He also noticed the water level was falling, now it was only just above his knees. The little people saw that Toby was getting disturbed. They threw more rocks and then tree branches into the stream until the water level was down to Toby's ankles. This made him very angry. He wanted to attack the little people. He felt irritated, angry, and critical of what the little people were doing. When he tried to move toward the little people, he found he was paralyzed.

Toby woke up in a panic and spent the morning wondering what the strange dream meant. He carried on reading the scroll and soon noticed that he resented certain people. When one of them did something that displeased him, he would be irritated all day, going over the incident in his mind. In council meetings he found himself still judging everyone and everything. He noticed how he listened to conversations and how judgmental he was. Some days he felt so angry that he would get headaches and tension in his shoulders. Then he would go off by himself to pray and clear his mind, but some times even prayer didn't work. Then he would get angry at himself. Still, he continued to read the scroll but it wasn't making much sense.

One day as he walked to the tribal chambers a child at play threw a small stone that accidentally hit Toby on the shoulder. Toby walked on, but he was furious. When he got to the office, it was locked because the janitor was late. The man had simply overslept, but Toby gave him a piece of his mind. Then he waited in the tribal chambers for two hours before the other council members showed up. By then he was steaming. It was one thing after another all morning. By noon he was thoroughly upset and went to his secret spot to pray, but sensing his prayers would be fruitless, he just sat there for an hour. At the afternoon council he felt resentful, angry, lonely and tired. He was belligerent at the meeting and said a lot of things he didn't really mean. Still he continued to read the scroll. That night he couldn't shake the stress and went to bed with a headache. He dreamt again of the little people throwing rocks, boulders, and tree trunks into the creek until it was only ankle deep. In the morning when he read the scroll, he felt there was a connection between the scroll and the dream, but he didn't see it clearly and spent another day gathering resentments and storing up anger. He still tried to pray, but his prayers were ineffective. He felt quite out of control.

Toby was troubled by the recurring dream and tried to figure out what it meant. Then he recalled that a woman in a neighboring village had the power to interpret dreams. He found her sitting in a rocking chair on the porch of her cabin. He handed her a gift of tobacco and asked for help in understanding his dream. She went inside her cabin and came out with a medicine pouch. Then she sent Toby into the woods to get a small bundle of cedar. She laid the cedar in a small circle and built a fire inside it. She put a pan on the fire and poured some roots and other medicine in it. She had Toby sit on the ground in front of the fire, facing west. She smudged him with sweet grass and then sat down facing north. Then she asked him to tell her the dream. As Toby spoke, the medicine smoke swirled around them. When he finished the story, she was silent for a long time before she spoke.

"The creek represents the power of the Great Spirit. When you stand in the power, you have wisdom, clarity, knowledge of God's will. This allows you to function in the world so that when you speak, the words are not your words, but the words of the Creator. When you decide something, it's not you who is deciding, but the Great Spirit working inside of you, who is deciding. It's not your intellect working, but the Intellect which runs the universe directing you. You automatically see all things through your love's eye. Even when you are verbally attacked, you will see that all attacks are a cry out for love, and then you will see people differently. This power flows inside of you and is always available.

"There are certain things that can block your access to this power. The power that blocks is also inside of you. This is what the little people were showing you. The first stone represents resentments. Whenever you have a resentment, you lose power. The second stone represents your anger. Having both resentments and anger will cause the power to decrease. Power always flows in the path of least resistance, just as water flows down the mountain.

"If the creek is flowing freely down the mountain and you are standing in the creek and someone upstream throws rocks in the creek, the water will not flow to where you are standing. If more rocks are thrown, soon you will only be ankle deep in power. Let's say you have anger boulders, resentment stones, judgemental logs, and you let them pile up. After that, let's say you remember to pray but you are only ankle deep in power so it may seem your prayers are not answered.

"Would it be more effective to ask the Great Spirit for an answer to a problem or to ask to have the blockages removed? If you pray to have the blockages removed, then you are standing in the answer and standing once again in the power. When you are angry at another person, you block yourself from God. When you ask God to remove the blockage, you will not attack the person—you will love him.

Each evening, clean up your stream. Get rid of any blockages to the power. Go to sleep as a peaceful warrior."

Toby had a real growing experience during the next three weeks. He recognized the value of having a clear mind. He became aware of the blockages created by his resentment, anger, fear, and self-pity. He began to see the good effects of self-examination and asking the Creator to remove blockages. He realized his relationships needed to be threesomes of himself, the other person, and the Creator. If he got upset or angry with someone, he needed to talk to the Creator first. He recognized that if he didn't clean up the garbage-thinking each day, he would carry it into the next day and it would block off the power.

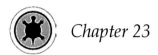 *Chapter 23*

A Visit from the Star People

Toby saw that the scrolls were having an effect on his life. He was no longer struggling with alcohol. As he changed himself by praying every morning, seeing conflict as a friend, and getting rid of garbage each evening, his personal life and relationships with the community began to go more smoothly. Now he had a new scroll about the powers of the north, the direction of wisdom.

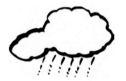

Reading Scroll Five

~ Use The Powers Of The North ~

Toby had never thought much about wisdom. He figured it was something you naturally got as you became older. As he was pondering the scroll, his hand touched the medicine bag hanging around his neck. He closed his eyes and could feel the bag pulsing in his hand. The quieter his mind became, the stronger the power became. He felt himself entering a new place in his mind. He squeezed the pulsing medicine bag harder until he sensed his whole body as a pulse, a heart beat. He let his mind get quieter. Suddenly, he felt himself entering a tunnel and falling. Frightened, he let go of the medicine bag and returned to his normal state of mind, feeling somewhat shaken. He decided to talk with the Elders.

In the meantime, he continued reading the scroll four times each day, facing north. One night after his reading he lay on the ground gazing at the stars. His hand came to the medicine bag and the sensation of power was there again. He squeezed the medicine bag harder, and as before, felt a pulse. Then he noticed movement among the stars. Four of them were getting bigger and moving toward him. As they approached, he saw they had the form of human beings.

"We are the star people. Your prayers have summoned us and we are here to help you." They looked like Indian people except they were the color of stars.

Toby looked at them for a long time. Finally he was able to speak. "I am a leader of my people and we are going through a difficult time. I am seeking wisdom, so I ask for help from the powers of the north. Can you tell me how to acquire wisdom?"

The first star said, "If you pray to the north, you will be given four freedoms: Freedom from fear, Freedom from hate, Freedom from self, and Freedom from knowledge."

The second star said, "If you pray to the north, you will be given insight, the ability to see within."

The third star said, "If you pray to the north, you will be centered during conflict."

The fourth star said, "If you pray to the north, you will be given the gift of intuition, the ability to see opportunity and avoid disaster."

Then the star people rose slowly back into the sky, and returned to their positions. Toby fell asleep.

He woke to sounds of birds singing and the smell of dew. He opened his eyes, thinking how he loved this time of the morning when all things seemed so peaceful and fresh. Walking back to his house, he recalled the visit of the star people. He had heard the old ones talk about the star people, but never thought he would actually encounter them.

The next week there was a meeting with some government officials who wanted to present a proposal to the council. At first, it wasn't very clear what the meeting was about. But after a couple of hours, it appeared that the government wanted to put a temporary nuclear waste dump on the reservation. They would pay millions of dollars that could be used for the tribe. There would be tremendous advantages to the tribe in education, jobs, and future funding possibilities. There were no dangers and the storage facility would be temporary, lasting for no more than 40 years.

As the government people continued their presentation, Toby's insides were in a turmoil. His internal radar system was screaming. When the meeting broke for lunch the council ate together and all of them were excited, thinking the dump would be a real break for the community. They focused on the economic advantages and how they would finally have money in the tribal treasury. Toby sat in silence. In the afternoon, the government presented campaign strategies with colorful posters, pamphlets and other persuasive literature designed to get the community's support.

The government people wanted the tribal council to present the idea to the community. They wanted to hear the response of each council member individually. One by one, the members expressed their support for the program. Toby was the only one opposed. "I know you see a great opportunity for the tribe in this proposal, but I cannot support it." He said this with so much conviction that everyone in the room was stunned. The tribal governor stated he would present the proposal to the community within the week and summarily closed the meeting.

That night as Toby read the scroll, he began to understand what the star people said about the gifts of the north. Throughout the next day, he sat in conflict and he stayed centered. He was not seduced by the prospect of material things and money. His internal radar system was on full alert. He knew the government proposal was not a good thing for the people.

At the next council meeting, a number of community members were present. Word had gotten around that the village would be receiving millions of dollars and they would all have high-paying jobs. Everyone listened carefully to the council members, who were practicing their usual politics, saying the right things to remain popular with the people. Toby sat in silence. The council decided to have the community meeting on Friday evening with a potluck so there would be a good turnout. The council spent the rest of the week planning what to say about the government proposal. Toby talked to the Elders and prayed to the powers of the north.

Friday night, the community center was packed. After the potluck supper, the council used the government materials to inform the community about the proposal. The people were excited and there were many questions. The council sat at a table in front of everyone and fielded the questions very well. Toby sat in silence. Finally, one of the Elders raised her hand. She asked why Toby was so silent and whether he had something to say. Toby's insides began to quiver. He sat for a long time and the room got very quiet. He picked up his Eagle feather and stood. He looked at all the people. He felt the medicine bag pulsing on his chest.

"Most of you I have known since I was a little boy. I have no secrets from you. Most of you watched me grow up and you watched me make my life's mistakes. I have hurt many of you, and you have also watched me hurt myself and my family. You watched me make a fool of myself and almost destroy everything that I love. You watched my bout with alcohol and the destructive path it took me on. So, in a way I am nothing.

"Despite all of this, I never stopped loving you, and I never stopped caring about my community and our land—our Mother

Earth. Now that I am sober, I love you even more and my respect for the Earth Mother is greater. These last few months of my sobriety, I have especially watched our children. I have really appreciated the support of my wife and family. So, it is for the children, my family, and our Mother Earth, that I speak.

"Our Mother Earth is alive. Would you pour poison into the veins of your mother? How much money would you need to store poison in your mother's heart? Suppose they told you, 'Let me store the poison for just a few years.' Would you do it?

"If your woman was still bearing children, would you let them store poison in her womb? What would happen to the children? Would you do this for money?

"Our land is our life blood. When the land is gone, so will our people be gone. We will disappear. What, then, will we tell our children? We did this for money?

"We are the keepers of the Earth. That is our destiny, assigned by the Great Spirit. He said to the red people, 'I make you to be keepers of the Earth.' We must think of the future generations, even about our children unborn. What are we leaving for them? Have we forgotten our spiritual ways?"

The room was completely quiet. Toby took his seat with tears rolling down his face. One by one, the community members stood up and slowly walked out of the room. The meeting was over. The council now knew where the people stood. They met the next day and sent a letter to Washington, refusing the proposal.

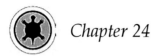 *Chapter 24*

The Six Powers of Interconnectedness

Toby sat at Maggie's breakfast table as he waited for the next scroll. The coffee was hot, the morning was fresh, and he felt close to the Creator. Maggie brought the scroll, and after a pleasant conversation, Toby headed for his favorite place by the water. The morning was so beautiful, he paused for a while just to watch nature. He closed his eyes and listened to the various sounds, then opened his eyes and focused on the many different colors. Closing his eyes again, he tested his sense of smell on the wind, identifying the fragrances of his surroundings.

Reading Scroll Six

~ Interconnectedness ~

Toby sat by the water and opened the scroll: "We are all connected." It was about community, but it reminded him of nature. He knew that everything in nature is connected in a balanced way. Nature thrives in harmony. But Toby had not considered how the various tribal organizations were connected. It seemed very simple, yet somehow difficult. As he thought about interconnectedness, he realized he didn't know much about it. He had heard the Elders talk about it some, but hadn't paid much attention. Toby decided to ask Tom Green, the medicine man, about it, and set off for his house. There he learned that Tom was away and wouldn't be back for another week. Toby continued to read the scroll and observe the community.

The following week Toby went to Tom and offered him some tobacco. He asked for help in understanding interconnectedness. Tom nodded and said he would help Toby gain this knowledge. Toby was to come back at ten that night, just after the moon showed itself above the horizon.

When Toby arrived, Tom had a fire burning in his back yard near a sweat lodge. Rocks were being heated for the sweat. On the fire a steaming kettle produced an unusual smell. The night was beautiful and Toby enjoyed the stars and watching the old medicine man who sang as he mixed the herbs. To Toby this was a mystery, but for Tom this was his comfort zone – working the Medicine, functioning in the Mystery.

Tom finished his preparations with a prayer to the Great Spirit. Then he turned to Toby. "Tonight I ask you to trust me. You must never discuss what will happen here with anyone without my permission." Toby agreed. Tom opened the door of the sweat lodge and invited Toby inside. The firekeeper placed the first rocks in the sweat lodge. The flap was closed and the heat increased rapidly. Cedar was sprinkled on the hot rocks and the space filled with its aroma. Tom started the prayers for the people. As water was sprinkled on the rocks, it sizzled into steam and the lodge became even hotter. When more rocks were brought in, Tom sprinkled them with the ingredients from the kettle and a very different aroma filled the lodge. Toby's body began to tingle. Tom spoke again. "Toby, you are going to the land of interconnectedness. This will help you lead our people. The Medicine I have poured will take you to the Unseen world, so you can see for yourself what interconnectedness is. You will be taken to the place of little people. When you get there, an Elder will meet you and he will explain and answer all your questions." Then Tom poured more of the brew on the fire.

Toby felt drowsy, but he was still awake. Soon, he sensed that he was shrinking. The lodge seemed to get bigger as Toby felt smaller and smaller. Then he was surrounded by a light beam. He was standing inside a cylinder of light and around it many paths of light extended in all directions. Toby sensed a force that seemed to be moving around him in a circle. Then he noticed another force circling in the opposite direction. Toby stood there in awe.

Toby heard a sound behind him. He spun around and there stood an Elder woman. "My name is Morning Star. I was sent here to assist you and to answer your questions." Toby asked her where he was. "You are in the center of an atom. You are at the center of all."

"In order for you to understand interconnectedness, you will see in a different way, opposite to what you normally do. You are conditioned to see the physical world, but not the spiritual world. While you are here, you will be able to see the spiritual world and also the physical world. If you roll your eyes up about fifteen degrees, a screen will appear in your mind. It will show you the physical aspect of your experience in the spiritual world. The sensations you feel, the cyclic forces, are orbiting energy fields called electrons and protons. The light you are standing in is the interconnectedness.

Morning Star told Toby to look at the screen. Toby rolled his eyes up, and Tom appeared, sitting in a lodge with his eyes closed. Morning Star continued to speak. "At this moment, we are experiencing the inner atom structure of the medicine man."

Morning Star suggested the two of them take a walk. "Which way?" asked Toby.

Morning Star replied, "Whatever path you choose."

From time to time as Toby walked through the atom field, he glanced at the screen in his head. He was leaving the body of the medicine man. As he reached the edge of the body, he sensed a change in the rotation of the energy fields. He entered the atom system of the air, but the path he was on was connected to the atom system of the atmosphere just outside Tom's body. He watched the screen as he moved from place to place on the path of interconnectedness. One moment there would be a tree. Then, as he moved, he would see a flower, a bird, then water and next another human being.

Even though the screen was displaying different objects and he was leaving and entering them, from the viewpoint of interconnectedness, it was one continuous system. When Toby saw this, he turned to Morning Star, smiling. He finally understood.

Toby asked Morning Star, "What is the interconnectedness made of?"

"There are six powers that make interconnectedness. They are love, intelligence, power, truth, principles, and life."

"How does this work?"

"When two people are standing next to each other, they are connected by truth. If one of them lies or is dishonest, the other will be able to sense the dishonesty. All words spoken must be aligned to truth. If you use good words, but the intent and meaning behind the words are dishonest, other people will be able to feel it. Words in themselves have no meaning, only the spirit and intent behind the words have meaning.

"In times of difficulty, you have direct access to these powers. You have direct access to the intelligence system, direct access to truth, direct access to love and direct access to principles. You get access to them either through meditation or by calming your mind. As is said, *be still and know.* When you are still, these forces will let you know. This is why the old ones say the answers are within you. When you are facing daily problems, don't focus on the problems, focus on the solutions. Learn to focus your attention on the stillness. After a little practice you will find this very practical. These powers are at your disposal, ready to be used."

Toby looked at Morning Star in bewilderment. She only smiled but then said Toby had learned and observed enough and it was time for them to depart. Toby felt himself slowly getting bigger. Soon, he was sitting next to Tom in the sweat lodge. They sang a song of thanks and left the lodge.

The next day, Toby read the scroll again and headed for the tribal offices. On the way, he noticed his outlook on the community had changed. As he walked, he felt the interconnectedness. Throughout the day he as he spoke with different people he was able to focus on the interconnectedness. He could see when people were dishonest and when they were confused.

During the tribal council sessions, he understood that every decision had consequences that vibrated throughout the community. He saw that mental health was connected to housing and housing was connected to the school and the school was connected to the council. This was so evident to him that he suggested having joint council and department head meetings. He saw the value of making decisions as a group for, if they could do it, the council would be more effective. Through the month, Toby's understanding of interconnectedness grew and he began to use the six powers to help him resolve tribal issues.

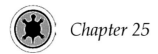 *Chapter 25*

Bringing Back the Cultural Ways

Maggie brought the next scroll one morning and reviewed the instructions with Toby once again. He was especially drawn to this new scroll on spirituality. Toby studied the scroll four times each day, just as he had been instructed. He began to look within himself. He questioned his identity as an Indian man and as a community leader. He began to see how much the Native leadership had adopted European ways.

As he studied the scroll, Toby thought it would be good for the council to consult with the Elders about bringing some of their own cultural ways back into the tribal government. He suggested an entire day's meeting and the council agreed. The Elders suggested spending the day on one of the islands, away from the normal business of the community. It took four large canoes to get the Elders, the council and their supplies to the island. When they were settled in, the Elders began to share their knowledge.

Reading Scroll Seven

~ *The Power Of Spirituality* ~

First, the Elder Joe Stone played the drum and sang a thank-you song. Then Joe Crow took an Eagle feather and prayed in his Native language.

Oh Great Spirit, whose voice I hear in the wind.

Hear us, for we are small and weak.

We seek your strength and wisdom today, as we meet to counsel in the old ways.

Without your guidance we are nothing.

Send the Spirits to help us with our difficulties.

Teach us to be responsible leaders and help us relearn the culture.

Open our minds to your ways so we look at our people with straight eyes.

Toby began the meeting by reading the scroll. Then he asked the Elders to say what they thought it meant. They sat in silence for a long time. Finally Joe Crow said, "We have waited a long time for you to ask us our opinion. We have been praying for many years for the leadership to come to us. So it is an honor for us to be here. We will talk to you about what our Elders told us about the leaders of the old days.

"The leaders of the old days were very dedicated to the people. They knew the only way to lead was to be spiritual themselves. They were in constant prayer and ceremony. They asked the Creator to help them with their decisions. They prayed before every meeting and before every decision. Each leader also knew the history and the importance of the culture. They knew the ceremonial songs. These leaders were very solid in the way they knew themselves, both their strengths and their weaknesses. They were not ashamed of their spirituality. Each of them tried to keep his or her heart clean.

"For leaders to be clear about their power, they should always know the answer to three questions. These questions are the keys to being connected with the spiritual world, which is where your power is. If you know the answers to these questions, you will be spiritually sound and will have access to the spiritual laws for guidance. If you do not know the answers to these three questions, you will feel disconnected, lost and afraid. If you know the answers, your prayers will go smoothly. If not, you may struggle with prayer. You may feel that the Creator is not answering. You may have a difficult time with focus. You will feel disconnected from people. You will want to be alone. You will want to isolate. Your heart may feel heavy. So listen carefully to what we have to say.

"The first question is: **Why am I?**

"Every leader must clearly know the answer to this question. What is your purpose? Knowing your purpose brings focus, concentration, and clarity. Clarity of purpose is the source of energy. It will wake up a problem-solving genius inside of you. You will attract people to help you. You will become very persuasive. Finding your purpose is the way to know what the Great Spirit's will is for you. If you cannot find your purpose, then start helping others, for the Creator's purpose for each of us is hidden in the seed of service to others.

"The second question is: **Who am I?**

"All leaders know their identity. They are clear about their self-worth. They are clear about their relationships with the Creator, with their community, and with themselves. They have strong personal values such as respect, commitment, resiliency, trust, loyalty, and balance. Leaders who know their identity also know their boundaries. The boundaries are healthy and they are spiritual. When your boundaries are clear, you say the things that need to be said. You quit people-pleasing. You do not react to fear. When people threaten you with their own stuff, you are able to tell which is yours and which is theirs. You develop a code of ethics and live by it.

"The third question is: **Where am I going?**

"Leaders are vision people. Each morning they ask the Great One, the Creator, to give them a vision and a direction, so they have a sense of God's will in every area of their lives. They carefully watch their thoughts during the day, for they know that we move toward and become like what we think. The direction of their lives is established by the Great Spirit.

"We Elders will come to the council meeting each morning to open the day with prayer. We will teach you the ceremonies and songs and show you how to use the drum. We have spoken."

The leaders sat in silence. Many of them felt ashamed because they now realized they were immature. They knew the council was not living the traditions. They knew the way they made decisions was part of the problem. They had been passing tribal resolutions, knowing they would not need to enforce them. They had been bad-mouthing one another and avoiding conflicts. They played favorites and gave jobs to their friends and relatives. Some knew they were doing things only for the advantage of themselves and their immediate families. The tribal governor and Toby gazed at each other for a long time. Then Toby noticed the sun was low in the sky and knew it was time for all of them to return to the village.

In the morning, the Elders came to the tribal offices to offer the morning prayers, but before they began, the governor asked Toby to read the paper he had read on the island. The council members nodded their heads in approval, so Toby read the scroll and then the Elders prayed. They continued doing this each day. Then the Elders began teaching the sacred songs to the council, in the evenings twice each week. The council started to change. They began to arrive on time for meetings. They started to listen, really listen. They began to avoid snap decisions. They started to talk to the people and ask for ideas. Toby carried on, reading the scroll at the council meeting each morning. The Elders continued to pray, and the council continued to change.

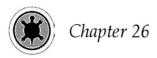 Chapter 26

Making Decisions for the Seventh Generation

M aggie and Jim sat by the shore fishing when Toby came for the next scroll. As they walked back to Maggie's place, Jim and Toby talked about what was going on in the village. Maggie gave Toby the scroll and went off to do an errand. Jim was talking about the old times in his tribe, telling stories he had heard from his grandfather. One of them stuck in his mind so he decided to share it with Toby. It is the story of the Eagle and the Mouse.

Jim's Story

"The world has two points of view. One point of view is from the mouse. The mouse has a world-view. When mouse gets up in the morning, all the grass is fifty times taller than the mouse and he has a hard time seeing. Every rock is ten times bigger than the mouse, so the mouse has obstacles to his vision. Every animal he encounters is a threat, so mouse walks about with fear. Any little dip in the earth is a major problem for mouse. He cannot step across even a two-inch gap, but must climb down one side and up the other. So, if you could hear mouse talk, he would say, "Oh my God, I can't see anything, everything I do is a struggle, life is so unfair, everyone is out to get me. How will I ever make it through the day?

"While mouse is anxiously going through his day, high in the sky is an eagle watching the same situation. Eagle is circling and listening to mouse's anxiety, turmoil and stress. Finally eagle shouts down to mouse, "Hey, mouse, lighten up! It may not happen as you fear it will happen. I'm seeing the same thing you are from another point of view. Your worry is meaningless. Lighten up!"

When Toby arrived at the council meeting, the Sparrowhawk family was arguing with some of the council members. Jim Sparrowhawk felt the council was unfair because they would not give his family money to pay their utility bill. It was an ongoing problem with this and other families. Many tribe members would get stranded somewhere and call the tribal office to wire them money to get back to the village. Many of them drank away their money, and would then demand help from the council, sometimes bringing their children along.

The Elders who had come to pray simply listened to this altercation. When all the council had arrived, they went into the meeting room and one of them lit some sage. Everyone smudged and the room got quiet.

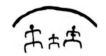

Reading Scroll Eight

~ Decisions Are For The People First ~

The Elder Luke began to speak. "A long time ago, our people knew how to fish together. Then, the white man got involved and started to bring us the fish in a box. For many years, our people have been eating fish out of a box. Now, we don't know how to fish. We must teach our people how to fish again. They don't think about taking care of themselves." After he said this, he sang a prayer.

The Elders left and the council talked about how difficult it was to respond to the people with their hard luck stories. They didn't mind providing assistance when it was legitimate, but when the people drank their money up and then demanded help, it was hard, especially when there were children involved. The tribe had very little money set aside for emergencies, but the people seemed to think the fund was unlimited and that they could demand money anytime they wanted it. If the council didn't respond, they would threaten recalls and spread gossip and rumors. It was hard to refuse help to people who drank up their money when their children had no food or clothes. And when they brought the children to the council meeting, it became even more difficult for the members to say no. The people had developed an attitude of entitlement. Their attitude had become, "You owe me." This caused them to further lose their skills and self-worth, so they became victims of this dependency.

Toby thought it would be helpful to share the latest scroll with the council. They agreed, so Toby read the scroll. The council knew in their hearts that it was right to make decisions first for all the people. They also knew the difficulties this new way might cause in their own families, who were used to being taken care of first. But they decided to try it for a month. They took a large piece of paper and drew the symbol of the scroll so they would be reminded about how to change their priorities.

Throughout the day, the council discussed each topic and then asked, "What decision can we make that will be of most benefit to the community?" When they discussed allocating some grant money, they could have fought among themselves and sent the money to places where their relatives worked, but instead they gave it to the tribal treatment center where all the families would benefit. As the week progressed, the council started to see how the new approach made decision-making easier. They could explain the reasons for their decisions to anyone who objected. They began connecting their decisions to the greater whole and to future generations. They started to ask, "If we make this decision, how will it affect the seventh generation?" They realized that every decision they made had consequences for the whole community. They began to see that each leader's decision had consequences for the entire community. If the director of the mental health department decided to give a raise to all his staff, it would cause problems in other departments. So they recognized that keeping each other informed would prevent many problems.

Each day the council met, they became more effective as leaders of the people. In the old days, they had bad-mouthed each other and gossiped behind each others' backs. It was a way to be popular with the people. But now they realized this backstabbing was hurting everyone. In the council meetings, they became more supportive of each other. As they saw more and more positive results, they developed into a unified council.

Eventually they realized they needed to share their growth with the people. "We are starting to act like leaders and the people may get suspicious that we are up to something. We need to communicate and educate everyone about our new standards of leadership." They would post a big board outside the council chambers to display the code of ethics by which the council was to be governed. And they would communicate the code, as it developed, in the tribal newsletter.

That afternoon, the bulletin board was put up with the first item in the code of ethics: **When we make a decision, the first priority is for the good of the People.**

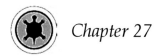 *Chapter 27*

The Power of Love Exists in the Heart

Toby received the ninth scroll and decided to go off by himself. As he was untying his canoe, Slow Turtle, the medicine man, came by. When Toby told him he was going to the island to pray and fast, Slow Turtle asked if he could go along. Toby said he would be honored.

Neither spoke as they paddled to the island. They simply enjoyed the water and the fresh breeze. On the island, Slow Turtle led the way to a sacred spot where his grandfather had fasted and prayed. There was a circle of rocks with a hole at the center. As they set up camp, Slow Turtle mentioned that each time his grandfather visited this place he returned changed, both physically and mentally. That night Toby read the scroll and thought about it. He watched the blazing campfire and the old man meditating, sitting with his hands out, his eyes closed, and a peaceful look on his face. Toby leaned against a rock, listened, watched, and felt full of peace. He had begun his fast.

Reading Scroll Nine

~ *Conflict Precedes Clarity* ~

Toby dreamt that smoke was coming from the circle of rocks. It seemed to be twisting as it rose. He sensed something controlling the direction of the smoke as it formed an arc to the edge of the circle. It was moving sunwise around the circle. When it touched a stone, the stone would turn white and start to glow. When the smoke had touched all the stones, the entire circle glowed with a bright light that seemed to have a feeling with it. Then the smoke drifted to the right and formed another circle. The smoke shone a light on it and Toby saw a circle of white stones with a circle of light inside that looked like an arena.

Soon, many little people appeared in both circles. Toby noticed that the people in both circles were identical to each other. Soon they started to talk and communicate with each other as if they were acting out a play or a story. They were acting out the same experiences but their words and actions were different.

Toby focused on the little arena with the spotlight and saw that the little people there were attacking each other verbally and that they seemed to enjoy the conflict. They called one another names and put each other down. Some of them were gossiping about each other. They were jealous and selfish. They were belittling, sarcastic, and treated each other badly. They teased in hurtful ways. They formed little cliques and plotted against one another. They were intentionally harming each other. Some were killing others, even their relatives. The married men and women were cheating on each other. The children watched the adults and very soon began acting in the same ways. The longer the drama went on, the worse it got. All their words and emotions were based on fear. The entire group was about to self-destruct.

Then Toby focused on the circle of white stones. The people there were having similar experiences, but when there was a conflict they formed a circle and prayed with an Eagle feather. As they held the Eagle feather up, the white light from the stones formed a beam of light that flowed toward the feather. When the prayer was finished, each person held the Eagle feather and spoke about how they felt at that moment while the others nodded respectfully. They were not necessarily agreeing, but tolerantly allowed the speaker to express him or herself fully. When everyone had been heard, they made a decision and moved on to the next matter. Toby saw that all the participants prayed each morning and that their main goal was unity, not attack. They chose to see good in each other and to forgive each other when there were difficulties. Periodically, the light from the stones flowed to the people.

Toby saw there were two ways to live. There were two ways to think. People could form a love-based system or a fear-based system. The dream continued and Toby saw that one of the people in the stone circle went off alone, built a small altar and began to pray. Soon the light from all the rocks responded and moved toward this individual who developed a special glow. As the glowing person returned to the circle, the little people stood in a line to shake hands. The glowing person reached the end of the line and started toward the other circle. As soon as she entered, the people attacked her in their usual way. The glowing person did not fight back, instead she concentrated on their heart area. This turned on a little light in their heart. It seemed she knew that looking at that special place in the heart would ignite the glow. One by one, she turned on the lights in each of the little people. The more they attacked her, the more she concentrated on their hearts and on what she said to them. Soon, they began to treat each other better. As they treated each other more kindly, small glowing pebbles formed a circle around them. As the little people continued to grow spiritually, so did the size of the pebbles. Soon they were sitting in a circle to deal with conflicts. They were praying with the Eagle feather and the light was flowing to them also.

Toby woke up and saw that Slow Turtle was still asleep and the fire was nearly out. He put some wood on the fire and, as he moved back toward his blanket, accidentally put his hand on one of the rocks from the circle. It was extremely warm. Toby touched each rock and found them all equally warm. He sat quietly until dawn.

Morning came on slowly. Toby began thinking about ending the fast. He looked around and noticed that Slow Turtle had left camp, probably to offer his morning prayer. As Toby was cooking breakfast, he heard the crackle of brush as Slow Turtle came back into camp. Toby turned to greet him and was startled to see a look of surprise on the old man's face. Toby jumped up and asked what was wrong. Slow Turtle simply beckoned and Toby followed him, mystified. They arrived at a quiet pond where the Elder silently indicated Toby should kneel by the water. Toby saw from his reflection that his hair had turned completely white. He fell back in fear and surprise. Slow Turtle explained that his grandfather had been changed in the same way. He returned to camp while Toby stayed by the water to pray.

In the afternoon when they returned to the village, Toby asked Slow Turtle to go ahead of him to explain to his wife and family. As he sat by the water, Nina came running toward him. They held each other in silence for a long time.

It didn't take long for the news to spread through the community. Next morning, as Toby approached the tribal offices, people were peeking around corners and out of windows, and the children stared with curiosity. Now Toby understood the scroll. As he studied it and worked with the people, he realized he only needed to remember the love in their hearts. Toby continued to grow in knowledge and wisdom.

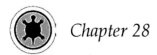 *Chapter 28*

The Community is Changing

At first, the council couldn't get used to Toby. Not only had his physical appearance changed, but his demeanor was so different that people stared. He seemed to have a circle of peace surrounding him. This attracted people, and they found he had become a very good listener. As Toby continued to read the scroll, things started to come together. He began to see that values are tools for resolving conflicts. Soon, Maggie approached Toby and offered him the next scroll, all about values. He accepted it gratefully and began to read.

Reading Scroll Ten
~ Use The Values Given By Mother Earth ~

When he approached council about the latest scroll, they readily agreed to discuss it. Toby explained the values and the council agreed to adopt them and to read them before every meeting as reminders of their code of conduct. They were written on the poster outside the tribal chambers. The council also agreed that after every meeting they would review their conduct in order to help themselves improve. Over the next few weeks, the people saw changes in the leadership. They didn't like all of them at first, but on the whole, it was getting better. In the old days when the people wanted something from the council, they had to yell and scream, but now the council listened, wrote things down, discussed things among themselves, and if they said they would get back to someone, they did it. But the most remarkable change was that the council was unified – there was no more back-stabbing or running each other down.

Then the council had the code of ethics posted in each building. They asked the schools to teach the values in all the grades. They asked the Elders to get involved and teach the values in the Native language. They designed a training program for all the tribal officials and insisted that they work to develop themselves according to the code. They had an artist paint the symbols in the tribal chambers to remind them of the values. Now, if the council could not agree, one of them would point at the symbols and request a few minutes of silence before they continued. In this way, the meetings became more effective.

During the following year, Toby was elected as tribal governor. The council continued to change and so did the community. As the leaders developed themselves in accordance with their values, the community members began to trust them. The council members continued to grow in wisdom and adopted more effective ways to relate to the people and to manage the business of the tribe. Many changes took place.

Leadership

First, the council turned their organizational chart upside down. They put the governor on the bottom, the council in the next tier, then the department heads, followed by tribal employees. The people were on the top. They called this *servant leadership* because the leaders were there to serve the people.

Then the tribal council made a commitment to fulfill the vision. They held a series of leadership workshops and insisted that all leaders attend them. They made the training available to anyone in the community who was considering a leadership position. And anyone who wanted to run for tribal office had to attend the leadership courses before submitting his or her name for nomination. The council realized that in the old days, leaders had been developed from childhood: they were nurtured by the Elders, they were taught to develop character. The people in the community watched the young grow into leaders so that eventually they were not just people to vote for, but people who had developed their characters and qualities. So, with the help of the Elders, a training program was created so high standards of leadership would be passed on from generation to generation.

The council arranged with the school to receive the names of any student from third grade onward who showed any natural leadership ability. Special classes and a multi-media collection of leadership materials were prepared. The students were invited to attend tribal council meetings and critique the council as part of their training.

Vision

Once the leadership was healthy enough, they called the entire community together and created a vision from questions that were asked of each community member.

What would our community look like if we were healthy?

Our Elders would be respected. The young people would be heard. Families would pray together and teach the culture to the young people. The people would speak the Indian language. The drum would be playing and the old songs would be sung by the young people. There would be family gatherings and the people would help each other. Young people would give their chairs to the old people. Ceremonies would be done for the people. There would be no domestic violence. Respect for women as sacred life-givers would be restored.

What would our leaders be like if they were healthy?

The leaders would really serve the people. If someone ran for a leadership position, he or she would be sober and would have attended the leadership training designed by the Elders. The people would know that their leaders got up early each morning and prayed to the Creator that their decisions would be for the greatest benefit of the people. A council of Elders would be formed to guide the tribal council during times of difficulty. It would be understood that each leader lived by the values of respect, trust, understanding, love, courage, tenacity, and would listen, think, and speak from the heart.

What do we want to see in our schools?

The tribal value system was incorporated in every area of the community. It was built into the performance evaluations of all tribal employees. It became part of the tribal school curriculum. The Elders gave frequent talks about traditional values all over the community. The community developed a career development plan for each child, from pre-school through adulthood. Language was taught K-12, Indian history was the primary course, the principles of math were taught by watching the aerodynamics of the Eagles' flight. Science was taught as an interconnected system of which the Creator was a part of all. Spirituality was a living part of the education system. Before each test, prayer was said and anyone who wanted to smudge with sage, cedar or corn pollen could do so. Many of the sports would be traditional games that taught honor and respect, not competition. The teachers would be taught to look at the Indian child as a bright, beautiful, inquisitive, spiritual child of the Creator.

What would our culture be like if we recovered some of the traditional ways?

Each morning the Elders would hold a ceremony at sunrise. Anyone who wanted to join could do so. The ceremony would be for the protection of the people. There would be ceremony for the children, and a puberty ceremony for the young men and women when their time came. At this time, the Elders would explain about womanhood and about manhood. They would explain about the responsibility of being an adult. The adults would relearn the old songs and teach them to the children. We would have family sweat lodges and teach the children about fasting. When we would do this, we would see the Earth about us begin to heal. We would understand that Nature is our teacher. We would watch her teach us about how to treat each other.

What would our environment be like if it was the way the Creator planned it?

We would see the powers of the four directions teaching us today, just as they did in the old days of our people. We would not throw our garbage on Mother Earth. We would not put poison in the water. We would not drain the Earth of her minerals, but use her in a balanced way. We would understand the traditional medicine and use it along with the modern medicine of today. We would take care of our Earth and show by example what it means to respect our Mother Earth.

Fruits of the Vision Book

The people continued to dream and vision. The Elders continued to talk about the old days and what their grandfathers and grandmothers told them. They talked about what was handed down orally, generation to generation. The people dreamed. Once the peoples' ideas were gathered, the council invited a group of community members to create a vision book. It was called *The People's Vision.* When they were finished, the vision book was shown to the people to make sure all their ideas were included.

Drugs and Alcohol

All tribal functions were free of alcohol and drugs. In the past, alcohol was a part of everyday life. After business meetings it was common practice to meet at the local tavern and drink. Many Indian conferences, both local and national, were well known as party times. Of course, what came with all of that was fighting, abuse, accidents, absent members, and bad decisions. But not any more. If a tribal official or employee traveled on community business, they were expected not to use drugs or alcohol. As the adults started to love this new way, the young people began to change their conduct as well. As the people started to get sober, families began to spend more time together. There were more sports and other activities attended by the whole community.

Feedback

For many years, the youth were not a priority, except when it came to using them to get grant money or if a person was running for a leadership position. Then the youth were important. Otherwise, what was said was only lip service. The people decided to give the youth a voice, a place where they could speak freely and people would listen to them.

Once a month, the youth were automatically scheduled to present their issues before tribal council. Once a month the agenda included time for the youth to explain to the tribal council what the issues for the young people were. The youth were allowed to voice solutions as well as input about other issues in the community.

When the youth said there was nothing for them to do in the evenings, the council formed a task force of youth to make recommendations. They were to come back in a month to present their findings. When the youth came back, they asked that the gymnasium be opened in the evenings. Another recommendation was to have a weekly basketball tournament between the adult men and the teenagers. They recommended a women's basketball tournament as well. They wanted the council to support other sports. They wanted a teen center. The council authorized the sports activities and donated an older building for a teen center, provided the teens would work to get the building supplies. The council paid one of the local carpenters to make sure the building changes were within codes. The youth set up their own guidelines on how the center would run. They created a youth management team to make sure the center was a safe and warm place for the teenagers to go to.

Elders

A council of Elders was formed. When the Elders started to meet in their circle, the community was invited to come and listen. Sometimes the old people would sit and tell stories. They were surprised at how many of the young people came to listen. Sometimes the Elders would let the people ask questions. The people would say, *Grandfather, Grandmother, talk to us about relationships. Talk to us about parenting. Talk to us about what your Grandfathers and Grandmothers talked to you about.* Although they spoke in English, the Elders started to use their traditional language. At first, just a few words, but as time went on they told the stories in the Indian language. The people began to understand the language again.

The Elders were once again available for council. The family structures were starting to be rebuilt. The Elders taught the young people to weave baskets and cut the trees to make them.

144

They taught the young men traditional games and how to build hunting weapons. They taught how to build canoes. A Great Learning was happening.

Training

Monthly seminars started to appear in the community to help members heal. These trainings were about co-dependency, alcoholism, relationships, conflict resolution, parenting, traditional culture and language. The community eventually developed their own TV station and used it for training and communication to the community.

Spirituality

The tribal leadership started each day with prayer. Soon the school was starting its day with prayer. Soon many of the families started their days with prayer. The Elders taught them how to conduct family circles once each week. Each family got an Eagle feather and committed to hold a family talking circle one night a week. On that night, the TV was turned off and the family did activities together.

Once a week, there was a community ceremony on the hill above the village. The people would come together, make some tobacco ties, put their prayers in the tobacco, tie the tobacco ties to a tree, and pray for the community. They asked the Creator to continue to help the people. As the weeks went on, more and more of the community members participated in the morning event, even though it was held at sunrise.

Culture

The drum group became very strong and had to form additional groups. Soon there was a drum group consisting of seven three-year-olds. The Elders started to teach the people the old dances and ceremonies. As the Great Learning took place, the rate of alcoholism decreased rapidly. It wasn't that the community no longer had problems. They did. The difference was in the way those problems were being resolved. The community was changing.

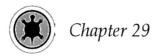 *Chapter 29*

A Story About the Healing of Conflict

The community was changing. The Elders talked about how conflict was resolved in the old days. There were certain clans or individuals who still held the knowledge of peace making. One day, two men came to the council for help with a long term dispute over some land. The council heard them out and sent them to the peacemakers. The peacemakers took them to a special, sacred place, a small peninsula with two large trees on the eastern and western shores. At high tide the men were seated beside each other, but one was to face west while the other looked to the east. They were both told to look at the trees, for the peacemakers didn't want them to make eye contact.

The peacemaker Elder working with the men knew our words can hurt people. Our words are like spears. When we speak them, we can hurt people. We can also heal people. The peacemaker knew the trees and the water are our friends. The water is for healing and the trees are a part of our breath. What we breathe out, the trees take in as food and return to us as new breath. Just as the trees make oxygen for us to breathe, they take on our hurt and return to us the spirit of healing.

The peacemaker lit some sage mixed with cedar and smudged both of the men as they sat there. Then he explained the rules. Only one man at a time was to speak. The peacemaker would give a talking stick to him, and the other man was to remain silent, even if what was said, was not true. When the first man was done, the peacemaker would give the talking stick to the other person. Then, only he could talk.

The first man spoke, clearly angry and hurt. The peacemaker continued smudging both of them. The angry words were carried on the smoke, then absorbed by the tree and the water below. His anger was not only about the land. He talked about how his father was an alcoholic and used to beat him when he was a child, about how he learned to stick up for himself because no one else would. Finally, he was done talking. The peacemaker, once again, smudged both of them with the medicine. The talking stick was given to the other and he started to talk also. He too, was very angry. He said how the land belonged to him. He needed the land to build his cabin on. He had just gone through a bitter divorce, and the tribal court gave his old house to his ex-wife—he had to have the land!! The tree also took on his hurt and the water carried it away.

When he was done speaking, the peacemaker smudged both of them, and returned the talking stick to the first man. This time, he was not so angry, for he now had some understanding of what was going on. Slowly, he started to feel compassion. There is a teaching that says, *when you are willing to change the way you are looking at something, what you are looking at changes.* When two people sit on opposite sides in a circle, they will see things differently. If they are willing to exchange seats, and look at it from the other person's point of view, when they return to their original seats, their opinions have changed. The talking stick was handed back and forth until the peacemaker could sense the hostility was over. The peacemaker knew that every disagreement has two parts. At first, people use words to hurt each other. Then, when both parties have begun to understand each other, there is an opening where healing can take place.

Now, the peacemaker had both men face each other. As they looked in each other's eyes, they could see they were brothers. Letting go of their anger let them see the love in each other. They came to an agreement about how they could share the land.

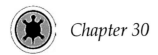 *Chapter 30*

The Warning

One morning Toby woke up early. He wanted to see Maggie, Jim and Grandfather and sent one of his sons to invite them. Over breakfast they reminisced about the many changes they'd seen in the community. They each shared their own understanding of what had happened. They agreed it was like living in a miracle. They recognized that the prophecies were coming true. Each of them was still surprised that they had been chosen as messengers.

The four felt very close. It wasn't like being brothers and sister but much deeper. They so strongly saw the meaning to life. They realized their primary purpose was to serve the Creator and help others. After breakfast, they moved outside and continued the conversation about how the community eventually had responded to the Elder's Teachings. Later that day Toby went to the islands to fish and relax. In the afternoon, just as he was about to fall asleep, he was startled by footsteps coming from behind. He spun around to see two unfamiliar Elders. They stood in silence. Toby heard more footsteps and Maggie appeared.

"We are Elders from the place of the Wisdomkeepers," they said. "We have one last assignment for you. Your people, Toby, are the keepers of the Eastern Door so it is only through you that we can reach the world.

"The world is on a destructive course," they continued. "If the world leadership continues to make decisions based on greed, fear, power, and control, Mother Earth will flip herself – meaning the north pole and the south pole will be reversed. In this way,

She will only let a few survive so She can start over. She did this already, one time in the past. When She decided to do this before, it was because the people had strayed off track. They forgot the Creator's laws and made up their own. Many of those laws were very self-serving. The people then were only interested in their own pleasure. Sick things became normal. Some people were enslaved and others were not considered human. The people started drinking alcohol and using drugs, which caused moral decay. There was in-fighting and power struggles. Families fell apart. Values were no longer important. Fear ruled their communities and governments. Abuse and violence became a way of life. The people were doing strange things, thinking they were so smart. They misused Mother Earth and they forgot how to pray. The Creator was no longer first in their lives.

"The Creator came to the place of the Wisdomkeepers and told us we needed to send the 'cryers' and warn the people that they were on a destructive path. For twenty-four years we went from village to village, warning the people. Most of them just laughed and wouldn't listen. In one small village, we found a family who was still living according to the principles of the Great Spirit. We told them to build a boat for themselves and the animals, because the Earth was going to flip and cause a great flood. While they built the boat, the other people laughed at them. But this family survived and everyone else died.

"Toby, we have given you the teachings that can show the people what must be done to break the cycle. The Earth is in critical times. We want you to write a book in the White Man's way, revealing what you have learned from our visit so that both our people and others may learn of the principles, laws and values that are helping renew your own community." Then the Elders built an altar and put a special medicine in the fire. They had Toby lean over the smoke while they sang. He closed his eyes and listened. He felt a stirring in his head and soon he remembered everything. Toby's heart was full of joy. Now things made sense.

The ceremony continued and the Elders continued to speak. "The people must wake up and look at what is happening," they said. "They must realize the importance of looking inside themselves. Each person must look within and listen to the small still voice. We cannot make them listen, for they are created with free will, with the ability to choose. Once again, in these times, the people have drifted off track. We have shown the world that a community can turn itself around by returning to the laws of the Great One. The people should recognize the signs. Poison is being put in the water, resources are being wasted, lives are being ruined by technology. The man is ignoring his family. He is greedy and not leaving things for future generations. His children are killing each other. The women are screaming in desperation about the children and the men are not listening. Children are having babies. Families are breaking up. New diseases are appearing and no cure is known.

"Tell him to look inside himself, for the Creator has written in his heart all the knowledge he needs to restore order. The only way he can get that information is through prayer. He must decide to let his world be ruled by God once again. These ancient scrolls and symbols are the keys. There is wisdom in each of them, which will whisper the secrets of healing.

"If we see enough leaders respond to this message, we will come again with more information. We know people are created with free will and will only change when they are ready. If the leaders don't respond, we will come again, but not until after Mother Earth has turned over. At that time all the resistors will be removed. Only the few people who have been living in the Creator's Ways will remain. If the leaders don't respond to this warning, we will wait and work with the chosen ones."

The Elders sat for a long time in silence. Then they slowly rose and walked down the trail. Toby and Maggie were in awe. They sat there quietly for a long time. The sun began its journey towards the western horizon. Soon, the full moon appeared above the eastern sea. Both Maggie and Toby were deep in thought. The night birds began to sing and the frogs were croaking. They sat in silence and peace. The moon continued its climb into the sky. After watching for a while, they stood up and headed back to the village.

So it is spoken. • *To all my Relations.* • *The People will live.*

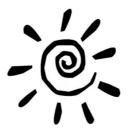

Epilog

Time flows onward beyond that day when the two Wisdomkeepers gave their warning in a last ceremony out on the islands. Toby, Maggie, Jim and Grandfather saw a lot of one another as the days and weeks became months and years. The community was slowly changing in a good way as a result of the Wisdomkeepers' visit. As a result of the teachings on the Ten Scrolls.

At first, a few community members came forward and asked if they could read one or two of the scrolls. In these early days, those who came forward in this way almost always felt something like an electric shock when they read a scroll. Each scroll talked directly to their hearts. At home, Maggie and Jim often served up a breakfast of fried salmon, eggs, toast and coffee to Grandfather, Toby, and a few community members who were passionately studying scrolls. On those days, the sharing was deep and joyful.

Little by little, the teachings of the scrolls also began to spread into the tribal offices and into tribal government. The people who were studying and who were moved by the teachings began to form a core group in tribal leadership and administration. Some days were still tough because the effects of alcohol, drugs, habits of abuse, and personal shame managed to assert themselves. But because there were people in tribal positions who were taking a look at themselves in active traditional healing, recovery from such bad days was quicker. On other days, respect, honesty, integrity and feelings of love could be felt in many of the tribal buildings.

One day in early autumn the four friends found themselves out on one of the islands. They had caught some fish and were roasting a delicious lunch at one of the spots many tribal people visited from time to time. After lunch a discussion about what was going on in the community naturally arose. Toby was struggling to verbalize some aspects of the change he saw taking place in the community. He said that some people were moving from some very negative ways, over into more positive and healthy ways.

Maggie became excited. After listening to Toby, she quietly reached into a traveling bag she brought along. With a mysterious smile on her face she brought out two drawings. Holding up one she said, "From this?" And then she held up the other one and said, "To this?"

Her companions studied both pictures and also became excited. There were some new words and ideas in the pictures but together they really nailed what Toby had been talking about. Where did you get these? they wondered out loud. But Maggie just smiled. The pictures showed a transition of how things were for some individuals as well as for the community, to how they were becoming or how they could be.

Jim produced a couple of thermoses containing local herb teas. The conversation continued as they sipped their hot beverages. Each could see that the unwell community roots of *anger, guilt, shame* and *fear* naturally gave rise to the unhappy, unwell behaviors symbolize by the trees in that drawing. They could also see that the unwell community soil of the first picture was showing signs of giving way to the healthier soil of *healing, spirituality, ceremonies, Native language, renewed cultural values, respect for the Elders' teachings, and the unity of interconnectedness* in the second picture.

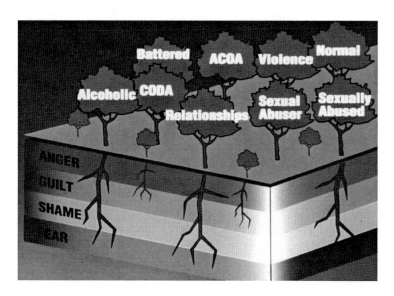

From This

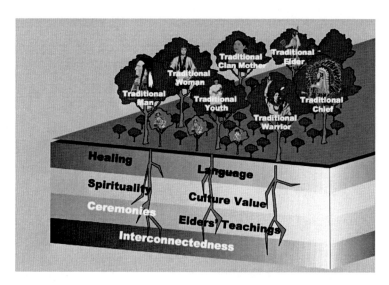

To This!

They could also see that there were very definite and tangible reasons for some of these positive changes. For example, there were now learning circles in a number of different local communities devoted to studying the scrolls in a traditional, ceremonial way. Some people who benefited from 12 Step alcohol and drug recovery now spoke openly of "working the Scrolls."

Other folks suddenly seemed to become interested in continuing their education in a nearby community college. The college was offering a Native studies degree with special focus on their own tribe's history. Some of the classes were taught by tribal Elders. Along with Native studies, people were studying and gaining very useful skills in writing, mathematics, science, technology, accounting, business, teaching and other core competencies. Learning all this along with both culture and healing made a lot of sense and led to jobs or further education at graduation.

Jim could see that the first signs of healing in this community were just coming into view. He was also trying to express something else. He saw the tangible changes taking place in the *seen* world, but what kinds of principles, laws and values were expressing themselves in the *unseen* or spiritual world?

Grandfather was quietly following the conversation and he, too, reached into a small bag and produced a drawing. He explained how he and some of the Elders had been visiting one another with renewed happiness and purpose from the time of the Wisdomkeepers onward. He revealed that he and some of his friends still lived by the principles, laws and values expressed in the Scrolls. Holding up his drawing, he said there is one deep root of positive change we think is happening.

One graphic was in the form of a triangle and showed a male human being at the very top of a grouping of other living beings, including a female human being. It was labeled "Ego." It meant that the man dominated it all, even superior to his own women.

Ego meant that it is all about him and that he thinks he is separate from, or outside the whole.

The other drawing was a circle enclosing all Creator's children as One within the whole. It was labeled "Nature," meaning that all life is part of, and subject to natural law. It was clear that the triangle symbolized the dominant Eurocentric view of the White Man on Mother Earth. It was also clear that the circle drawing expressed the Indian or indigenous view of Mother Earth. In the Native view, different beings offered different gifts, but all were fundamentally equal in the eyes of Great Spirit.

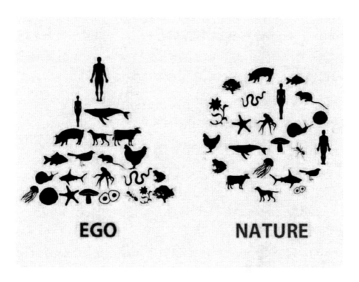

The companions were moved because these two graphics by themselves told the story of really different viewpoints. One viewpoint, presented as a triangle, is today destroying the Mother Earth and is the subject of the Wisdomkeepers' Warning. The other, represented by a circle, is the way of Indian people and is the road of healing, hope, unity and forgiveness – the way of wellbeing and sustainability. Grandfather said he saw the beginnings of change from the Ego-view to the Nature-view taking place. Everyone wondered where grandfather had gotten the drawing. But grandfather just smiled.

The sun was sinking low in the sky. The four friends broke camp and headed back to the mainland. Jim, Maggie and Grandfather returned home but Toby took a roundabout walk back to the tribal offices. He reflected on the drawings and how they related to leadership and governance in his community.

He knew that tribal governments had been modeled after the U.S. government since the Indian Reorganization Act of 1934. This meant that the triangle drawing had been forced on them when in fact their own way was that of the circle drawing. This was one source of their struggle.

He knew there was a lot of work to be done in moving back to their own indigenous ways of governance while at the same time living within a Turtle Island (North America) that had become dominated by the disharmony of the triangle drawing.

He knew it would take well people, strong in their own Native traditions, and also capable in the ways of mainstream society, to bring traditional Native leadership back into the indigenous communities of both the United States and Canada.

Entering the tribal building Toby caught an aroma of ceremonial cedar and sage and heard laughter coming from one of the meeting rooms. Peeking in he saw a traditional talking circle of many men and women working with one of the scrolls. A participant was energetically creating a colorful mind map on the white board from comments flowing out from the circle.

Toby listened for a while and knew the journey they had been discussing out on the island was well underway in the community. He knew they were at the beginning of a long journey. He offered joyful tears and a humble Thank You! to Creator. Heading home to his own family, he sang a traditional song of gratitude.